KOREAN BEAUTY SECRETS

A PRACTICAL GUIDE TO CUTTING-EDGE SKINCARE & MAKEUP

KERRY THOMPSON & COCO PARK

KOREAN BEAUTY SECRETS

A PRACTICAL GUIDE TO CUTTING-EDGE SKINCARE & MAKEUP

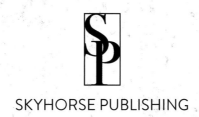

SKYHORSE PUBLISHING

Skyhorse Publishing books may be purchased in bulk at special discounts for sales promotion, corporate gifts, fund-raising, or educational purposes. Special editions can also be created to specifications. For details, contact the Special Sales Department, Skyhorse Publishing, 307 West 36th Street, 11th Floor, New York, NY 10018 or info@ skyhorsepublishing.com.

Skyhorse® and Skyhorse Publishing® are registered trademarks of Skyhorse Publishing, Inc.®, a Delaware corporation.

Visit our website at www.skyhorsepublishing.com.

10 9 8 7 6 5 4 3 2 1

Library of Congress Cataloging-in-Publication Data is available on file.

Cover design by Kerry Thompson and Coco Park
Cover Photo by Pedram Navid

Print ISBN: 978-1-63450-651-9
Ebook ISBN: 978-1-5107-0119-9

Printed in China

For my sister, Liz, for being the best sister, best friend, and best support system anyone could hope for, and also for doing the dishes every day for the past three months.

— Kerry

For the Park family, whose support made not only this book, but my career possible, and the Rush family for always being there, no matter what. My Nanny Jo (Nola Carmel), for not only introducing me to glamour, but for encouraging me to seek out the bright lights of the city and not be the country mouse like ole' Squashbug. I love you all so very much.

Yakoke. Chi hollo li.

— Coco

CONTENTS

KOREAN BEAUTY SECRETS

A PRACTICAL GUIDE TO CUTTING-EDGE SKINCARE & MAKEUP

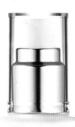

PART 1
KOREAN BEAUTY CULTURE

Korean cosmetics culture dates all the way back to the Three Kingdoms Era (57 BC—668 BC), when it was believed that an attractive outer appearance could carry over into the inner self, creating a culture that attracted both men and women to cosmetics. Women wore makeup to enhance the appearance of health, making rouge and lipsticks from botanical ingredients such as safflower. The aristocrats were oftentimes inspired by the cosmetic stylings of the *kisaeng*, who were entertainers for the royal courts of the Goryeo and Joseon Dynasties.

These days, the tradition of emulating the looks of entertainers holds fast, as skincare and makeup trends are carried over into the mainstream by Korean actresses and pop stars. These beloved celebrities achieve cult-like status amongst their fans, who rush to imitate their style. If a popular celebrity spends just a few seconds in a K-drama using a particular product, or is even simply photographed using it, it just might spark a frenzy, causing the product to sell out across the country. With the growing international popularity of the "K-Wave," or *Hallyu* movement, these stars, looks, and products are washing ashore just about everywhere. Modern-day Korean beauty culture is now easily one of the biggest influencers in the worldwide beauty industry.

Western cosmetic companies have been looking to Asia for product inspiration for years. The most obvious example of this is in BB creams, which took the North American market by storm in 2012. BB creams had already been a staple in the Korean market since 2005, and enjoyed soaring popularity thanks to the numerous celebrity endorsements they received. Since the rise of BB cream, Korean beauty products have received increasingly more visibility in Western media, and there are more people than ever embracing the skincare and makeup offerings brought to us from South Korea. It's not hard to understand why: there is a lot to love about them.

The number of savvy consumers combined with the high prioritization of skincare and makeup as essential purchases in Korean culture has ignited and cultivated a highly-competitive pressure-cooker of innovation. This creates a huge advantage for consumers—the rivalry means cosmetic companies are driven to produce remarkable, high-quality products at rapid speeds. These offerings are frequently packaged in unique and appealing ways in order to stand out from the competition and attract the attention of discerning consumers, and many of the products are competitively priced.

Additionally, though the testing process for emerging ingredients in South Korea is extremely rigorous, new discoveries are still brought to market more quickly and frequently. Sometimes these new ingredients prove to be gimmicky fads, a phenomenon that occurs in the beauty industry in all parts of the world. But that's not always the case—one trend we've noticed in the Korean beauty industry is the tendency for cosmetic companies to quickly adopt discoveries that are made in the biomedicine sector. There are many ingredients that are unique to the Korean cosmetic market that are making their way into formulas in other parts of the world because there is some promising, legitimate scientific research to back the claims.

The high quality, innovation, competitive pricing, and visual appeal of Korean cosmetic products have put the industry in a position to disrupt the beauty market in other parts of the globe. We embraced it long ago, and we haven't looked back. We are both enjoying the best skin of our lives, and it is our belief that Korean cosmetics can work for anyone

It was an intimidating world when we first started out, and there were many new product categories we had to familiarize ourselves with. We've learned so much since we began this journey, and now we want to help you uncover what makes Korean makeup and skincare so unique, as well as guide you through the process of assembling a Korean-style skincare routine and putting together your own Korean-inspired makeup looks. Whether you're a seasoned fan of Korean cosmetics or complete newcomer to the world of K-beauty, we hope that you'll discover something in these pages that will change your beauty routine for the better!

— Kerry & Coco

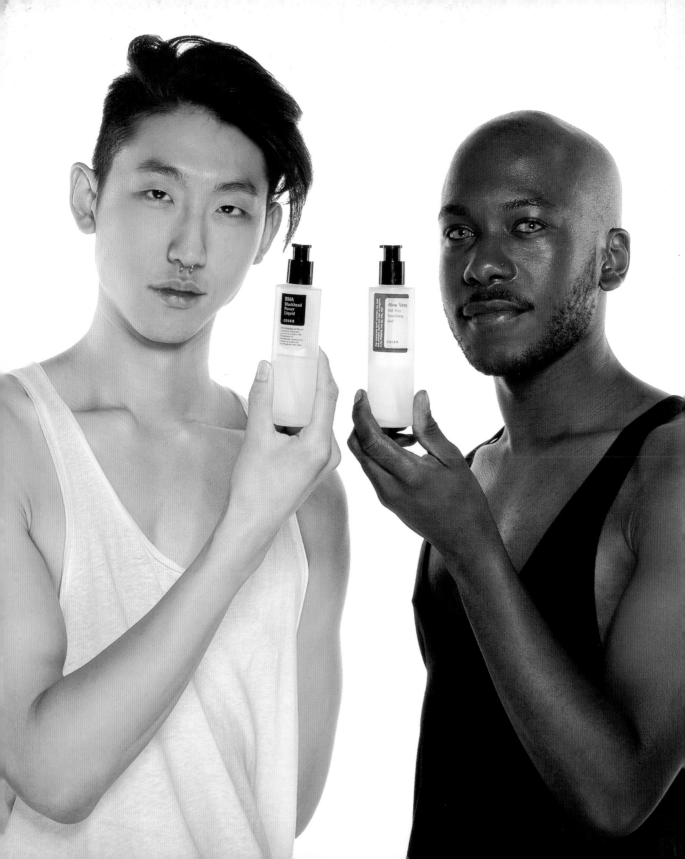

If you're new to shopping for Korean cosmetics, looking for recognizable brand names can be a good starting point for making purchase decisions. That's not to say that a product needs to be manufactured by a huge conglomerate to be good; in fact, many of our favorite products are produced by smaller, independent beauty brands. But having some brand names in mind can help expedite the process of seeking out new products, and it also makes scanning the vast array of Korean cosmetics online and in-store a little less overwhelming.

There is an incredibly large number of beauty brands in South Korea, some of which have been around for decades, and many more that have materialized over the past several years. In the pages that follow, we'll take a look at these brands, how they're positioned, and where you can find them.

BRAND FAMILIES

Although there are more than one thousand cosmetic brands in the Korean beauty space, the biggest share of both domestic cosmetic sales and beauty exports are dominated by two leading cosmetic and personal-care conglomerates. Both Amorepacific and LG Household & Healthcare boast impressive beauty portfolios that contain a range of top-selling brand names spanning multiple price points and venues.

AMOREPACIFIC BRAND FAMILY

In the world of Korean beauty, Amorepacific dominates the space. You might recognize quite a few of the names in their brand portfolio, since many of them have already permeated European and North American markets, and can even be found for sale in global retail chains such as Sephora, Target, Neiman Marcus, and Nordstrom.

LG HOUSEHOLD & HEALTHCARE BRAND FAMILY

Not far behind Amorepacific in terms of market share is LG Household & Healthcare, which is a subsidiary of the LG Group. Outside of Asia, the LG Group is largely known for its electronics manufacturing, but in South Korea, LG is the second largest producer of cosmetics and personal care products. Like Amorepacific, LG Household & Healthcare has an array of highly acclaimed brands in its beauty portfolio, which cover a variety of price points and venue types.

AMOREPACIFIC

Sulwhasoo	H E R A	IOPE
HANYUL 韓律	LIRIKOS	LANEIGE
ARITAUM	primera	make ON
ODYSSEY	MIREPA	Mamonde
eSpoir	illi HANBANG BIO 一班	TEEN: CLEAR
ETUDE HOUSE	HAPPY BATH natural	innisfree

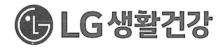 LG 생활건강

The history of

su:m 37°		O HUI
belif believe in truth	VDL	ĬSA KNOX
BEYOND	VONIN	LACVERT
시작, 아름다운 전설 Sooryehan	THEFACESHOP NATURAL STORY 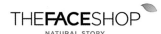	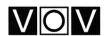 V O V
CathyCat COLORIST	KACHET	FROSTINE'S FROST THE LIMIT

BRAND CATEGORIES & STORES

To better understand how customers shop for and interact with Korean beauty brands, it helps to understand where they're sold. In the United States, the beauty market is generally divided into two categories: drugstore brands and department store brands. There are a handful of exceptions that fall outside of these venues, but for the most part, American beauty brands are either one or the other.

By contrast, Korea has a number of venues where brands may be sold, and some brands may be sold in more than one venue type. For example, there is a lot of crossover between department store brands and those that are sold door-to-door. Let's take a closer look at the different types of beauty retail venues and what makes them each unique.

ROAD SHOPS

Ah, Korean road shops! What are they? Why are they called road shops? And where can we find them? "Road shops" are, quite literally, shops on a road. Each road shop is dedicated to a specific mass-market brand or brand family, and price tags span from low to mid-range. If you want to compare road shop prices to those of Western brands, Revlon at the bottom of the cost scale all the way up through MAC would be a close analogy.

Some road shop products roughly equate with what North America and Europe sees as drugstore or high street brands, while others are more on par with mid-range department store lines. I say "roughly" because in actuality, though Korean health and beauty stores and hypermarkets may carry items from some of these labels, a majority of the in-person sales for these brands takes place in the dedicated road shops.

Examples of road shop brands include *Missha, The Face Shop,* and *Banila Co.*

HEALTH & BEAUTY STORES

Much like drugstores elsewhere in the world, Korean drugstores, such as Olive Young or Boons, offer a large selection of cosmetics from an extensive assortment of brands. But there is one major and enviable difference: the cosmetics truly dominate the store space. Imagine a drugstore that feels more like a Sephora, with a couple of aisles of snacks and medicine thrown into the mix. That's the Korean drugstore experience!

Additionally, the beauty products and brands available in this setting are, on the whole, higher-end than those you might find in a U.S. drugstore. For these reasons, this retail setting can be more accurately described as a "health and beauty" store rather than a drugstore.

Price points span from economy to mid-range, similar to the price ranges for many of the road shops. In fact, some of the brands found in health and beauty stores can also be found in their own, dedicated road shops, while others can also be found online or in hypermarkets.

Dr.Jart+, Skin79, and *Sooryehan* are examples of brands available in Korean health and beauty stores.

DEPARTMENT STORES

Department stores in Korea offer all of the allure of chic, sophisticated, shopping as first-tier department stores in other parts of the world. The stores are vast and upscale, carrying clothing by high-fashion houses from all over the globe, as well as high-end cosmetics by domestic and international labels. The Korean beauty brands sold in department stores are of the luxury, high-priced variety.

Sulwhasoo, The History of Whoo, and *Su:m37* are all examples of Korean brands you would find in a department store setting.

HYPERMARKETS

Hypermarkets, for those who aren't familiar with the term, are large superstores that contain both a department store and a supermarket. Hypermarkets are far more economically priced than top-tier department stores. SuperTarget in the U.S. or Carrefour in France would be close equivalents of a hypermarket in Korea, such as E-Mart or Lotte Mart. These stores usually have a fairly large selection of cosmetics from economy to mid-range price points. Many of the brands sold in hypermarkets are also sold in brand-specific road shops and health and beauty stores.

Some brands you might find in a hypermarket include *Illi, VOV,* and *Iope.*

DOOR-TO-DOOR

The door-to-door cosmetics market is alive and well in South Korea. The sales methods are very similar to those used for door-to-door beauty sales in the U.S.: sellers either go door-to-door, host parties in their home, or set up a pop-up boutique in their neighborhood. But the key difference in Korean door-to-door sales is the caliber of the brands offered through this channel—many of them are the same, high-end luxury beauty brands found in Korea's top-tier department stores. There are also quite a few road shop and drugstore brands that are included in this sales method.

O-HUI, Isa Knox, and *Makeon* are examples of brands with a door-to-door sales force (as well as a presence in department stores, road shops, hypermarkets, or health and beauty stores).

LIST OF KOREAN BEAUTY BRANDS

With new Korean cosmetic companies emerging daily, it's impossible to keep up with them all, but we've put together an extensive list of cosmetic brand names to help you spot Korean cosmetic lines as you shop online and in stores all over the world. This list includes brands from every price point, from the sensibly economic to the luxuriously decadent.

3 Concept Eyes	BBIA	CathyCat	Davi
3W Clinic	Belif	Charm Zone	Dermalift
23 Years Old	Benton	Chica Y Chico	Dewytree
A'Pieu	Berrisom	Chosungah 22	Diaforce
Acwell	Beucle	ChungYoonJin	Doctorcos
A.H.C.	Beyond	Ciracle	Donginbi
Amorepacific	Botanic Farm	Clair's	Dr.G (Gowoonsesang)
Anskin	Brilliant	Clio	Dr. Oracle
Aritaum	BRTC	CNP Laboratory	Dr. Jart+
Aromatica	C20	COSRX	Duft & Doft
Banila Co.	Caolion	Cremorlab	ElishaCoy
Baviphat Urban Dollkiss	Carezone	Danahan	Elizavecca

Enca	Isoi	Mizon	Skin Ceramic
Enprani	Jaminkyung	Moonshot	Skin Factory
eSpoir	Kachet	Naexy	The Skin House
Etude House	Klairs	Nature Republic	Skin Miso
The Face Shop	Kocostar	O-Hui	Skin79
Freeset	LacVert	Odyssey	Skinfactory
From Nature	Laneige	Papa Recipe	Skinfood
Giverny	Leaders Clinic	Peripera	Skylake
Goodal	Leejiham (LJH)	Petitfe	SNP
Graymelin	Lei Lani	Primera	So Natural
Gwailnara	Lindsay	Pure Heals	Sooryehan
Hanskin	Lioele	Purebess	Su:m37
Hanyul	Lirikos	Purederm	Sulwhasoo
Hera	Lotree	ReDNA	Teen:Clear
The History of Whoo	The Lotus	REGENcos	TonyMoly
Holika Holika	Makeon	Rojukiss	Too Cool For School
I'm From	Mamonde	The Saem	Tosowoong
Illi	May Coop	Scinic	VDL
Innisfree	Mediheal	Secret Key	VOV
IOPE	Milkydress	Shara Shara	Welcos
IPKN	Mirepa	Sidmool	Whamisa
Isa Knox	Missha	Skin & Lab	WondeRuci

PART 2
KOREAN SKINCARE

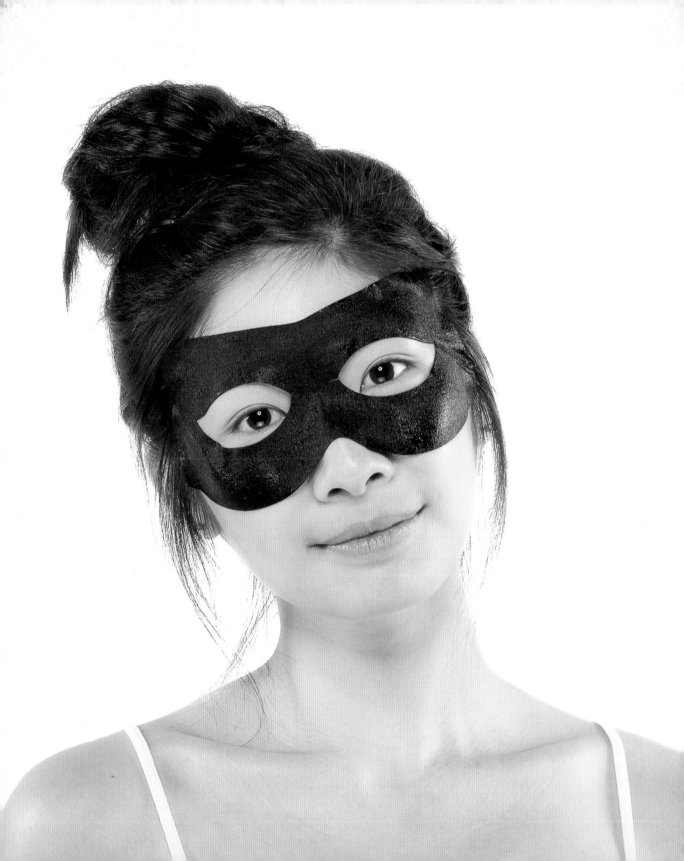

First things first—let's talk about what makes the Korean skincare approach so different from what many of us are used to. There's a common misconception that using Korean products is solely what makes a skincare routine "Korean." While that certainly helps, the origin of your products is only one small piece of the larger picture. In fact, it's possible to build a Korean influenced skincare routine without specifically using Korean skincare products at all! That said, there is an abundance of decadent, interesting, and effective products offered by the Korean skincare market, and you'd be missing out on a lot of the fun if you skipped out on them entirely.

There are many values and perspectives at the heart of the Korean skincare philosophy that make this approach so effective. Here are some of the primary distinctions of Korean skincare:

EMPHASIS ON HEALTHY SKIN RATHER THAN MAKEUP

South Korea's beauty industry is enormous, spanning both skincare and cosmetics. But far more money is spent on skincare products than on cosmetics, a result of the very smart cultural philosophy that beauty begins with healthy skin.

The ideal state for skin in Korea is dewy, clear, smooth, resilient, and luminous. You can get a more nuanced understanding of what exemplifies a perfect complexion in Korea by understanding some of the recently emerging terms used to define this optimal state. For example, *chok-chok* is a word that describes skin that is bouncy and moist; and *taeng-taeng* is used to describe skin that is firm and smooth.

For a majority of people around the world—including South Korea—this optimal complexion doesn't come naturally. It's something that must be worked toward with a consistent, effective skincare routine, and in Korea, that goal is worked toward diligently and passionately.

LAYERING & CUSTOMIZATION

In the United States, the standard routine tends to be a three-step process of cleansing, toning, and moisturizing. More skin-savvy women may have a four-step routine that also includes a serum. In contrast, a Korean skincare routine can have anywhere between five and twelve steps in the morning and evening. It seems excessive by comparison, and it may even sound like it would overwhelm the skin with moisture. But it's not overwhelming, thanks to the tendency toward lighter formulations of Korean products, which lean more on water and humectants to provide moisture than they do on emollient oils and occlusives. There is actually a solid logic behind such an elaborate, multi-product approach.

One advantage is the ability to customize your routine based on your skin's daily needs. If you know you'll be spending a lot of time in a dry environment one day and a humid environment the next, it's easy to adjust your skincare to accommodate those environmental changes.

It's also easy to customize a Korean skincare routine to treat specific skin concerns such as acne, aging, or hyperpigmentation. Having a multistep routine composed of light layers means you can have multiple products in your lineup that are each designed to provide targeted treatment for skincare concerns. If you have more than one skincare concern—and most people do—you can layer on individual serums that are each fine-tuned to effectively treat a specific concern, rather than having to rely on a product that tries to do it all. Additionally, having individual products to treat these concerns means that once your concerns change, you're not replacing your entire routine—you're replacing a single product.

FOCUS ON HYDRATION

Skin hydration is a key component of the Korean skincare approach. Hydration refers to moisture from water, as opposed to oils, and the idea is that hydrated skin is healthy skin. Well-hydrated skin functions better, and in the long term, it's more resistant to outside factors that cause aging. In the short term, hydrated skin appears fresh, resilient, translucent, and smooth.

Even though many Korean moisturizing products are domincated by watery and humectant ingredients, there are also wonderfully emollient oils and occlusives in a multitude Korean formulas. Those products are often designed to be applied later in the routine, in order to seal in the beneficial hydrating ingredients and the skin-plumping humectants.

EVEN SKIN TONE

Nearly every brand based in Korea has at least one skincare line devoted to "whitening." There are many misconceptions outside of Korea regarding this phenomenon, but first things first: no, these products do not bleach your skin. From an ingredient standpoint, the word "whitening" in the Korean beauty landscape is interchangeable with with the word "brightening." Whitening products are designed to even out skin tone and address hyperpigmentation due to the overproduction of melanin in damaged areas of the skin.

The ingredients used in mass-market whitening skincare products specifically target discolored areas either by exfoliation, which helps expedite the creation of new, healthy skin by increasing the rate of cell turnover to reveal newer, healthier cells, or by inhibiting the enzyme tyrosinase, which controls melanin production and causes hyperpigmentation in areas of the skin that have been damaged. This also includes the lightening of skin that has been tanned by the sun, which is, in fact, a form of sun damage. It just so happens to be a form of sun damage that has been embraced as a beauty standard in many parts of the world over the past century.

Interestingly, the first and most visible signs of aging in Asian women aren't lines or wrinkles—they are hyperpigmentation and dullness. The ideal healthy complexion is skin that is smooth, hydrated, even-toned, and luminous, and most products labeled as "whitening" can help anyone achieve this state, including deeper skin tones.

HIGHLY PRIORITIZED SUN PROTECTION

As important as the desire for an even skin tone is the emphasis on sun protection. Again, suntanned skin is damaged skin, and in Korea, a suntan is not the beauty goal that it is in other parts of the world. This is a very advantageous view when it comes to anti-aging. Sun damage, in addition to elevating the risk of skin cancer, is also the primary cause of visible signs of aging such as lines, wrinkles, and uneven skin tone.

Because sun protection is such a high priority in Asian markets, a lot of effort has been made to produce highly effective, cosmetically elegant sunscreens in a broad selection of formulas including creams, mists, gels, and essences. Furthermore, there is a lot of value placed on broad spectrum protection in Korean formulas—meaning these sun-protection products tend to be highly effective against both UVB and UVA rays.

The primary distinction between UVB and UVA is that UVB rays are responsible for sunburn, while UVA rays are responsible for cancer and premature aging. I find it helps to think of them as UVBurn- and UVAge-rays.

COMMON QUESTIONS

Do I have to follow all the steps?

There can be anywhere between five and twelve steps in a typical Korean-style skincare routine. It takes a bit of trial and error to find the right combination of products for your skin, as well the number of products you find personally ideal and, most important, sustainable. The most successful skincare routine is the one you can actually keep up with on a daily basis. For some, this will be only five steps, but for others, who have more skin concerns or who may (like myself) simply enjoy the lengthy, self-indulgent ritual, twelve steps could be just the beginning.

Product application typically goes in order from the thinnest product to the thickest—though it's important to consider other factors when building your own routine, such as pH-dependent ingredients (e.g., alpha-hydroxy-acids) or specific brand recommendations.

Is a Korean skincare routine time consuming?

Though it sounds like it would be a lengthy process, a multistep skincare routine doesn't have to be. A routine can be completed in ten minutes if it doesn't include products that require a wait time, such as a sheet mask or AHA treatment, either of which can add another fifteen to twenty minutes.

Is a Korean skincare routine expensive?

A Korean skincare routine is only as expensive as you want it to be. There is a huge range in terms of price points—skincare products can be priced as low as $8 and as high as over $600 for a moisturizing cream. But a large part of the appeal of the Korean skincare world is the high quality of the products, even those sold at lower price points. You can easily assemble an effective, luxurious Korean skincare routine composed of several products for less than $100.

Can I use non-Korean products in a Korean-style routine?

Contrary to popular belief, you don't need to use Korean products exclusively in order to benefit from a Korean-style skincare approach. You can achieve wonderful results by using whatever you have at home, or have access to in your particular part of the world.

Korean skincare products are wonderful, but the routine's approach is about much more than the geographic origins of your moisturizer. The Korean skincare philosophy is about prioritizing your skin as your most important beauty asset, focusing on moisture, and building a highly customized routine of light, hydrating layers that target specific skin concerns.

WHAT WE'LL COVER

The goal of this section is to supply you with all the tools you need to get started with a Korean-style skincare routine. In this section we will:

1. Assess your skincare needs
2. Examine skincare ingredients
3. Identify product types and categories
4. Build a skincare routine
5. View examples of skincare routines

With this information, you'll be able to confidently research and shop for Korean skincare products that will lead you to the smoothest, most luminous, and hydrated skin of your life!

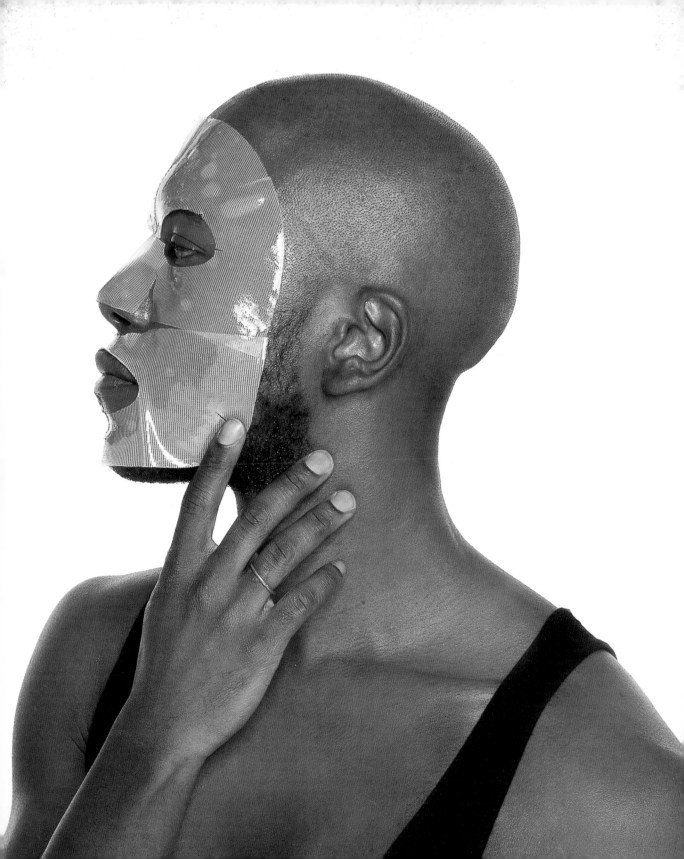

In this section, I'll be walking you through the process of determining your skin type and identifying skin concerns. Assessing your skin is the first and most crucial step in building any effective skincare routine.

Your skin can change over time, so it's important to do a skincare assessment periodically. Factors such as age, hormonal changes, lifestyle patterns, medications, medical conditions, and weather can all impact your skin, so it's possible that products that once worked wonders for you are suddenly not meeting your needs. Season changes are a great time to reassess your skin.

SKIN TYPE

Skin type is determined by how much sebum your skin naturally produces on its own. The amount of sebum your skin produces strongly influences not only how oily your skin might appear, but also how quickly your skin loses water, and therefore, how quickly it becomes dry. Your skin type can be normal, dry, oily, or combination.

To determine your skin type, wash your face and then wait an hour. Don't apply any skincare products after washing your face—doing so will interfere with your skin's normal state, and the idea here is to get an understanding of your skin's moisture and oil levels when it's left to its own devices.

Once the hour is up, it's time to observe! Examine your skin, and decide which of the following profiles is your best match.

NORMAL

Normal skin is skin that is balanced in terms of moisture. It produces enough natural oil to feel smooth to the touch and retain enough water that it stays moist, but not so much oil that it can be seen on the surface. Normal skin does not necessarily mean "perfect skin," but you tend to have fewer skin issues than many of your peers.

Your skin type is normal if:

- Your skin does not appear shiny or oily
- You skin does not feel tight or overly dry to the touch
- There are no obvious signs of flaking
- You have very few, if any, enlarged pores
- You tend to have very few acne breakouts, and those you do experience are minor

Normal skin benefits most from proper cleansing and moderate moisturizing. Hydrating toners, emulsions, and face oils are ideal for maintaining the enviable state of your skin.

DRY

Dry skin is characterized by an underproduction of sebum, which makes it less smooth to the touch and also prevents your skin from retaining the amount of water needed to keep it optimally hydrated.

Your skin type is dry if:

- Your skin feels tight
- You skin feels dry to the touch
- Your skin appears dull
- Any fine lines or wrinkles you may have appear more pronounced

Dry skin can also sometimes be indicated by:

- Flaking
- Red patches
- A textured appearance

It's important to note that sometimes people mistakenly believe they have dry skin, which is a skin type, when they are actually experiencing *dehydrated* skin, which is a skin concern. The difference is that dehydration is a temporary state that causes rapid water loss due to damage to the skin's natural protective barrier. This moisture barrier damage is generally brought on by outside factors. Additionally, it's possible (and actually common) for skin to be both dehydrated and oily. Dehydrated skin can be remedied in a few weeks and, with vigilance, kept away indefinitely once it's repaired.

By contrast, dry skin is dry even if the natural barrier is intact, because it's simply not producing enough sebum on its own. It is the long term state of your skin rather than a temporary condition that has a long term remedy.

Dry skin benefits most from multiple layers of hydration in the form of light, hydrating toners, humectant-based serums, and emollient face oils with a thicker, more occlusive cream layered on top to seal in the moisture.

OILY

Oily skin is characterized by an increased amount of surface oil caused by an overproduction of sebum. Oily skin tends to be visibly shiny and slick to the touch.

Your skin type is oily if:

- Your face is shiny with visible oil, especially at the end of the day
- Pores appear enlarged in some areas
- You experience frequent acne breakouts or blackheads

People with oily skin are often tempted to over cleanse with harsh, drying ingredients, or even avoid moisturizing altogether. This may seem to help in the short term, but in the long term, this can cause oiliness to worsen. These approaches make you more susceptible to a damaged moisture barrier, which would cause even more surface oil to emerge, and presents the risk of becoming a vicious cycle.

Instead of stripping skin with harsh cleansers and scrubs, switch to using an oil-based cleanser in conjunction with a gentle facial cleanser in the evening, and the same gentle facial cleanser on its own in the morning.

And don't skip out on moisturizing—oily skin still needs hydration. Just avoid the heavier creams, and stick with light emulsion formulas and watery, gel-based creams. Oily skin needs more humectant moisturizers, and fewer or no occlusive moisturizers.

COMBINATION

Combination skin is oily in some areas while being dry in others. One of the most common patterns for combination skin is an oily T-zone (forehead, nose, and chin) and dry cheeks, though combination skin can occur in other patterns as well. Keep in mind that minor differences in skin are normal; true combination skin has pronounced differences in oil production from one area of the face to the other.

Your skin type is combination if:

- It's noticeably oily in some areas while dry in other areas
- Pores in oily areas are enlarged
- Oily areas are more frequently prone to blackheads and acne breakouts
- Dry areas are prone to dry, red patches or flakiness

If you have combination skin, look for products that have "balancing" in the name or description of the product. These products are designed to keep your oily areas under control without drying out the rest of your skin. Light layers of hydration are key for combination skin because they provide moisture for dry areas without weighing down oily areas. Additionally, if the differences between your dry and oily areas are extreme, it can be beneficial to use different product types on contrasting areas of the face.

SKIN CONCERNS

"Skin concerns" describe a condition or occurrence outside of your skin's natural moisture levels. Acne, hyperpigmentation or red marks, aging, and dehydration are all skin concerns. The best way to identify your skin concerns is to think about what struggles you've had with your skin consistently over the past three months. This is enough time to identify an ongoing concern and distinguish between something that needs to be addressed and something that may have been a one-off, short term issue. Short term issues should be treated as well, but when investing in an entire skincare routine, looking at the big picture will bring you the most value.

ACNE

Acne is one of the most common skin concerns, as well as one the most complex skin conditions to care for. It can affect any skin type—even dry skin—though it's most commonly seen in oily and combination skin types. Acne can manifest as blackheads, whiteheads, closed comedones, cystic acne, or some combination of the above. While the occasional minor breakout is normal and common, those who are truly acne-prone suffer from frequent, consistent, moderate to severe breakouts.

Acne can be caused by multiple factors such as genetics, hormones (caused by pregnancy or even hormonal birth control), climate, product sensitivities, or a damaged moisture barrier.

There are a wide variety of cosmetic ingredients that treat acne symptoms. We'll look at some of those specific ingredients when we get to building your routine. It's important to note that some people are more responsive to certain treatments than others, so finding the right combination of ingredients to effectively combat acne can be a bit of a trial-and-error process.

Acne often occurs in conjunction with other skin concerns; hyperpigmentation and sensitivity are common additional concerns for acne sufferers.

Note: *Those with moderate to severe acne should visit a dermatologist or general practitioner, as sometimes acne can be a symptom of a larger medical issue such as PCOS or another serious condition. Additionally, doctors can prescribe stronger medication such as retinoids, antibiotics, or hormone supplements for acute acne cases.*

WRINKLES & FINE LINES

Aging is inevitable, therefore making wrinkles and lines the most common skin concern of all—it's something that everyone has to contend with at some point in their lives. Some people begin to see fine lines appear in their twenties, while others may not see any significant lining until well into their forties. The rate of aging varies widely for people, and is influenced by factors such as genetics, environment, sun exposure, and lifestyle choices. Although there are many causes of aging that are out of our control, there are also a number of steps that can be taken to delay their onset or lessen their severity.

Consistent skin hydration, sun protection, and proper cleansing are key factors in delaying the onset of wrinkles. It's ideal to begin these practices in the teen years, but it's never too late to start. If you're worried that you've missed the boat by neglecting your skin into your 20s and 30s, don't be! You may not have had a head start, but beginning a diligent skincare routine now will certainly slow the arrival of wrinkles that may form in the future, and diminish the intensity of the lines that have already appeared. It's far easier to prevent the signs of aging than it is to reduce them once they appear.

DEHYDRATED SKIN

Dehydrated skin is skin that is parched because of an inability to hold water. This condition happens when your skin's natural protective barrier, often referred to as the "moisture barrier," is damaged. Skin is composed of multiple layers, with the protective, outermost layer being the stratum corneum. This layer is also what is commonly referred to as the "moisture barrier." It's composed of dead, flattened cells called keratinocytes, which are continuously shed and replaced by newer keratinocytes and held together by fatty acids, ceramides, and sebum. Together, the sebum and keratinocytes act as a waterproof barrier that effectively keeps water in the skin and prevents bacteria, irritants, allergens, and other microorganisms from penetrating it. This surface layer of skin is slightly acidic, and can have a pH ranging from 4.0 to 7.0. Healthy skin tends to have a pH of 4.7 to 5.5, while higher pH levels are often accompanied by sensitivity, acne, and even eczema.

When the moisture barrier is compromised, skin is left unprotected and begins to experience water loss. This leaves skin susceptible to dryness, irritation, stinging, redness, sensitivity, and acne. Moisture barrier damage can also cause an increase in sebum production as the body tries to repair what's been done. Additionally, the sebum your skin produces in its damaged state will be more visible on the surface, since there are more openings between cells for it to escape through when the barrier is compromised. If you've ever had skin that's simultaneously dry and oily, it's the result of a weakened moisture barrier struggling to correct itself.

There are many things that can cause damage to the moisture barrier. Common causes include:

- Overexfoliation
- Using cleansers or other skincare products with an alkaline pH (higher than 7.0).
- Cleansing too frequently or vigorously

- Sunburn
- Windburn
- Side effects of oral or topical medications
- Medical conditions

Dehydrated skin can manifest differently from person to person. Signs that your skin may be dehydrated can include:

- Extreme dryness, especially if sudden
- Sudden, pronounced appearance of wrinkles and fine lines
- Resistance to the absorption of skincare products
- The onset or an increase in skin sensitivity
- The onset or an increase in occurrences of acne breakouts, eczema, redness, flushing, or contact dermatitis
- Crepey and/or flaky patches, particularly around the eyes, nose, and tops of the cheeks
- Skin feels oily on the surface, but when touched or rubbed beneath the oil it feels thin, dry, and papery

Dehydrated skin can be frustrating to deal with, but with patience and the right skincare products, it can be easily corrected. The best remedies for dehydrated skin are gentle, low pH cleansers, and moisturizing products with humectant, emollient, and occlusive properties. The Korean skincare approach of product layering is actually quite ideal for addressing dehydrated skin, since it follows a pattern of light, hydrating layers of moisture followed by more emollient and occlusive products to seal that moisture in.

Once the moisture barrier has been repaired, many people find that other skin conditions they thought were separate concerns, such as acne and skin sensitivity, disappear as well. It can take anywhere from one to four weeks to heal a damaged barrier, so patience and consistency are important!

PH TIPS:

- Aim for cleansers that have a pH of 5.0 to 5.9 — this is the ideal range. A pH of 6.0 to 7.0 *can* be acceptable (pure water is 7.0, which is neutral), but lower is generally better, particularly for dehydrated or sensitive skin.
- Most cleansers don't advertise their pH in their literature or product packaging, but you can test it at home with a pH strip. They're very inexpensive and can be found on Amazon, eBay, or at your local drugstore.
- When measuring the pH of your cleanser at home, mix the cleanser with a bit of water. This will give you the most accurate picture of what the pH of the cleanser will be when it reaches your skin.
- If you can't pH test at home, you can always try contacting the manufacturer and asking about the product's pH level.

SENSITIVITY

Skin sensitivity is a complex skin concern that can be caused by a number of things. Some people have naturally sensitive skin, others may have sensitivity as a result of other skin conditions such as rosacea, allergies, a compromised moisture barrier, or as a side effect from another product in their routine (prescription retinoids, for example).

Skin sensitivity can manifest in a number of ways, including redness, flushing, or a burning sensation when certain skincare products are applied. It can also coincide with frequent contact dermatitis, eczema, or even acne. Sensitivity levels can vary widely in terms of severity.

Sensitive skin can be difficult to work around but, with patience, it's possible to find effective products that work for you. Recommended treatments for sensitive skin include gentle, low-pH cleansers without harsh surfactants, and an avoidance of skincare products that contain fragrance or alcohol. Regular application of gentle, hydrating skincare products, and sun protection is essential for the care of sensitive skin.

DULLNESS

Dullness is exactly what it sounds like—it describes skin that lacks brightness and has a lackluster appearance. It's often accompanied by an uneven skin texture, which only contributes to an overall drab appearance. It most commonly occurs with dry or combination skin types, and is caused by a build-up of excess dead skin cells.

Thankfully, this is a condition that is easily remedied. With exfoliation, consistent sun protection, and key skin-brightening ingredients, you can get your youthful, luminescent glow back in no time. In fact, the Korean skincare world has an insane number of products dedicated to this very purpose.

UNEVEN TONE / RED MARKS / HYPERPIGMENTATION

Uneven skin tone, hyperpigmentation, and red or brown marks left behind after a pimple has disappeared are all very common skin concerns caused by an over-production of melanin in a particular area. These marks and patches can be triggered by a number of things including acne, wounds, hormonal changes (especially pregnancy), or sun damage. Forms of discoloration can affect people of all ages for a host of reasons, but for many women, uneven skin tone and hyperpigmentation are the first and most visible sign of aging.

When the discoloration is caused by acne or a healed wound, it's often referred to as post-inflammatory hyperpigmentation (PIH) or, in some cases, post-inflammatory erythema (PIE). These types of spots can worsen if the area is picked at or if the preceding pimple was popped—so keep your hands away from that breakout, no matter how tempting it may be! PIH and PIE can also be worsened by infection, sun exposure, or additional injury to the area.

Some forms of discoloration are more easily dealt with than others, but all forms of hyperpigmentation can be improved upon and often completely remedied with the right skincare products. Many of the ingredients designed to treat dullness also do a great job lightening skin discolorations, and once again, the Korean skincare market has a lot of product ranges to offer when it comes to correcting melanin-related skin concerns.

NEXT: SKINCARE INGREDIENTS

Selecting the right products for your skin becomes infinitely more fruitful when you understand what the ingredients are and what they do. In this section, I'll be highlighting and describing many of the more prevalent ingredients found in skincare products and specifically, Korean skincare products.

TYPES OF MOISTURIZERS

Most of us know that moisturizing is essential for an effective skincare routine, no matter what your skin type may be. But what many do not realize is that not all moisturizing ingredients are the same—there are actually three separate classes of moisturizers: humectants, occlusives, and emollients.

A good moisturizing product, whether it be a cream or an emulsion, will usually have some combination of all three categories of moisturizing agents in addition to other beneficial skincare ingredients. Understanding the distinctions between classes of moisturizing ingredients can make all the difference in selecting the right products for your skin type.

HUMECTANTS

Mmmm. Humectants. If I had to choose a favorite class of moisturizers, it would probably be these little workhorse hydrating molecules. Humectants have the ability to attract, absorb, and hold water from nearby sources, like the deeper layers of your skin and, in very humid climates, the air. Applying humectant ingredients to the surface layers of your skin provides much needed moisture, and because most humectant molecules have the ability to hold more than their weight and water, you'll also benefit from a short term plumping effect that visibly smooths out fine lines and lessens the intensity of deep wrinkles. Consistent use of humectant-moisturizing ingredients can also slow the development of wrinkles in the long term.

Another reason to love this category of moisturizers is that there are many humectant ingredients that also offer additional skincare benefits. Honey and aloe vera are great examples; both ingredients provide anti-inflammatory, antioxidant, and antimicrobial effects in addition to their hydrating properties. Alpha-hydroxy-acids (AHAs) such as glycolic acid, lactic acid, and malic acid are another great example. All of those ingredients are highly effective, naturally-derived chemical exfoliators, and they also happen to fall into the humectant category. However, it's important to use caution with AHAs—using these ingredients too frequently or at very potent levels can damage the moisture barrier, which ultimately leads to dryness—the exact opposite of what we want from our humectant ingredients. But when used properly, you get skin that's hydrated, fresh, and bright.

If you're looking for a humectant that you can really go to town with, choose a product that features mild, soothing humectant ingredients, such as aloe, honey, hyaluronic acid, or plain-old glycerin.

In the world of Korean skincare, you'll find humectant moisturizing ingredients in a broad spectrum of creams and emulsions as well as serums, essences, and ampoules. Humectant ingredients also tend to be the primary constituents found in sheet mask essences, which is why sheet masks have such instant, visible effects on the smoothness and moisture levels of the skin.

Common Humectant Ingredients:

- AHAs (e.g., glycolic acid, lactic acid, malic acid, etc.)
- Aloe vera
- Glycerin
- Honey
- Hyaluronic acid
- Soluble collagen
- Urea
- Hexylene glycol
- Butylene glycol
- Propylene glycol
- Sugar alcohols (sorbitol, glycerol, xylitol, etc.)

OCCLUSIVES

Water loss is the primary reason for dry and dehydrated skin, and is something that is experienced by most people to varying degrees. People with healthy but naturally oily skin experience less water loss because their natural oils prevent water from escaping. Those of us with dry skin produce less sebum, so water loss tends to be a bigger problem. Water loss is especially problematic for sufferers of eczema, excessive flakiness, and extra dry patches, all of which can cause water loss and worsen with dryness. It's a very frustrating spiral! Fortunately, this is where occlusive ingredients can rescue us.

Moisturizing agents that fall into the occlusive category provide moisture by creating a physical barrier over the top layer of skin that prevents water loss and therefore, prevents dryness and all of the annoying effects that come with it. If applied to dry skin, occlusive ingredients won't moisturize much on their own—though they might provide some smoothing emollient effects. The true power of occlusives are experienced when they are applied over wet skin, or in conjunction with humectant ingredients. When used in this way, occlusive ingredients help dry skin receive maximum hydration benefits by preventing the water from escaping our skin.

Common Occlusive Ingredients:

- Beeswax
- Fatty acids
- Fatty alcohols
- Lanolin
- Lecithin
- Mineral oil
- Paraffin
- Petroleum
- Plant-based butters (e.g., cocoa butter, mango butter, shea butter, etc.)
- Silicone
- Stearates (e.g., glyceryl stearate, PEG-100 stearate, etc.)
- Vegetable-based waxes

EMOLLIENTS

Emollients are moisturizing ingredients that fill in the gaps between skin cells and smooth flakes, which not only makes skin appear smoother, but also makes skin softer and increases its flexibility. Emollients also possess some occlusive properties, preventing water loss through the skin, though generally not for as long or as effectively as a true occlusive can. The most visible property that sets emollients apart from occlusives tends to be the consistency—emollients are thinner and far more spreadable than ingredients commonly categorized as occlusives.

Many emollient ingredients provide some form of skin nourishment, since a number of them are plant- or animal-based oils. Most of these oils possess antioxidants, and many also boast anti-inflammatory and even antimicrobial properties. Oils also contain fatty acids, which help to strengthen our skin's natural protective barrier. This is especially helpful for those suffering from dehydrated skin conditions.

Common Emollient Ingredients:

- Plant-based oils (e.g., almond, argan, coconut, jojoba, olive, passion fruit, rosehip, etc.)
- Animal-based oils (e.g., emu, horse, mink, etc.)
- Glycerides
- Polyisobutane
- Squalane
- Squalene

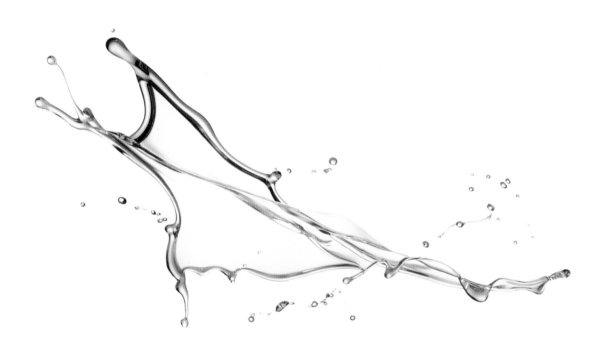

INGREDIENT GLOSSARY

There are thousands of skincare ingredients in existence. Fortunately, we don't have to know every single ingredient in existence to make good skincare decisions. A relatively small percentage of those ingredients actually appear frequently in skincare product formulas, and I've chosen to focus on more frequently seen ingredients in Korean skincare products that also bring the most value. The ingredients in this glossary all have some ability to improve and maintain skin quality, ranging from antioxidant properties, to spot-lightening abilities, to anti-aging help.

I've divided this glossary into four categories of ingredients commonly found in Korean skincare products:

- Conventional
- Experimental
- *Hanbang*
- UV filters

CONVENTIONAL

These are ingredients that can typically be found not only in Korean skincare products, but also in skincare formulas from all over the world. These ingredients have staying power because they've been time-tested and have some amount of scientific evidence that supports claims of efficacy for varying skin concerns.

Adenosine
Anti-inflammatory, wound-healing, and assists in regulating healthy cell function.

Alpha Hydroxy Acid (AHA)—Glycolic Acid, Lactic Acid, Malic Acid
A chemical compound that acts as an exfoliant, promotes cell turnover, and possesses humectant properties. Can be naturally occurring or synthetic.

Allantoin

Anti-inflammatory, wound-healing, emollient properties.

Aloe Vera

Antioxidant, anti-inflammatory, antibacterial, humectant properties.

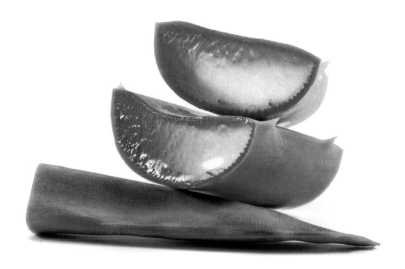

Amino Acids / Peptides

Anti-inflammatory, promotes collagen and elastin production.

Arbutin

A skin lightening agent derived from wheat, pears, or the bearberry plant, often used in spot lightening and brightening treatments.

Ascorbyl Tetraisopalmitate

A stable form of vitamin C, which provides antioxidant, brightening, anti-acne, and anti-aging benefits.

Azelaic Acid

Anti-inflammatory, antibacterial, compound used to treat acne and skin pigmentation issues.

Betaine Salicylate

A salicylic acid and betaine compound, which performs as an exfoliator as well as an anti-acne and antimicrobial agent. It's a gentle alternative to salicylic acid, which is a highly regulated ingredient in South Korea.

BHA—Salicylic Acid

Anti-inflammatory, antimicrobial chemical exfoliant used to treat acne and hyperpigmentation. Can be naturally occurring or synthetic.

Caffeine

Antioxidant and anti-inflammatory ingredient which can temporarily reduce redness and under-eye puffiness by constricting blood vessels.

Ceramides

Lipids that help repair and strengthen the skin's natural barrier system.

Charcoal

Highly absorbent carbon material which absorbs excess oil and impurities, sometimes used in deep cleansing and acne treatments.

Clay

Absorbent mineral used to absorb excess oil and impurities, often used in acne and pore refining treatments.

Cocoa Butter

Antioxidant-rich, plant-derived lipid which moisturizes and prevents water loss.

Collagen

Protein with humectant properties, usually appears in the form of soluble or hydrolyzed collagen. Provides hydrating and temporary skin-plumping effects.

EGF / Oligopeptides

Peptides composed of amino acids. Anti-inflammatory, promotes collagen and elastin production.

Glycerin

Humectant ingredient that provides hydrating and a temporary skin plumping effects.

Green Tea

Anti-inflammatory, antioxidant used in anti-aging formulas as well as treatments for sensitive skin.

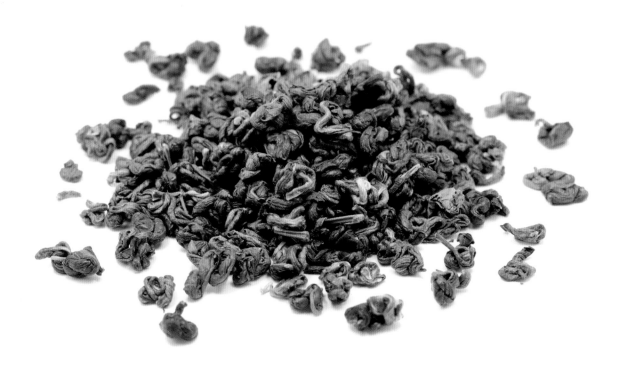

Honey

Anti-inflammatory, antimicrobial, antioxidant rich humectant ingredient with emollient properties, often used in formulas for treating dryness, acne, and skin irritation.

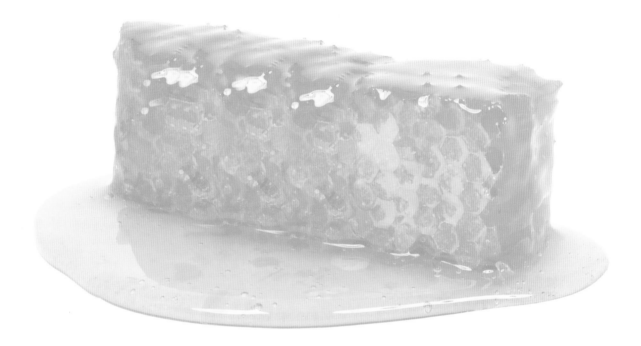

Hyaluronic Acid

Highly effective humectant ingredient which provides hydration and temporary skin plumping effects. Sometimes appears as *sodium hyaluronate.*

Lactobacillus Ferment

A probiotic in the lactic acid bacteria group with antioxidant, anti-inflammatory, and antimocrobial properties.

L-ascorbic Acid

Common form of vitamin C, which provides antioxidant, brightening, anti-acne, and anti-aging benefits.

Licorice Root

Anti-inflammatory and gentle skin-lightening ingredient often used to treat redness, dullness, and skin discoloration.

Mango Seed Butter

Antioxidant-rich, pant-derived lipid which moisturizes and prevents water loss.

Morus Alba / Mulberry Extract

Antioxidant extract which contains the skin-lightening compound, arbutin. Used to treat skin discoloration.

Natto Gum

Rich antioxidant source derived from fermented soybeans.

Niacinamide

Vitamin B3, maintains and improves skin elasticity, treats and prevents acne, lightens hyperpigmentation, prevents and treats redness.

Plant-Based Oils

Plant-derived, fatty acid-rich lipids with emollient and antioxidant properties. Can also be anti-inflammatory and/or anti-microbial. Includes oils such as argan, olive, meadowfoam seed, green tea seed, sunflower, camellia, and marula.

Propolis

Resinous material produced by bees. Antioxidant, anti-inflammatory, antibacterial, and antifungal, used in formulas for treating acne or irritation.

Retinoids: Retinaldehyde / Retinal, Retinol, Retinyl Palmitate

A form of vitamin A with the ability to regulate cell turnover, as well as prevent and reduce fine lines, wrinkles, and acne.

Rice Bran Extract

Anti-inflammatory, vitamin E-rich, plant-derived oil, rich in fatty acids, emollient properties.

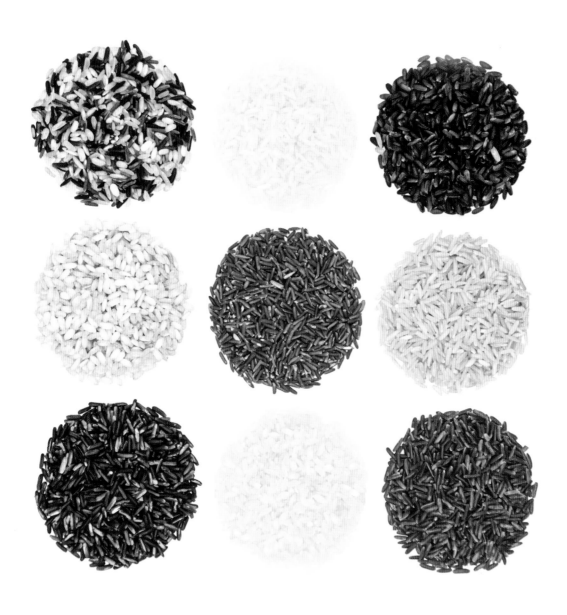

Shea Butter

Antioxidant-rich, plant-derived lipid that moisturizes and prevents water loss.

Squalene / Squalane

A lipid derived from shark liver, olives, wheat bran, rice, or sugar cane with emollient and antioxidant properties. Squalane is a more stabilized form of squalene.

Tea Tree Oil

Antimicrobial, anti-fungal essential oil, effective for treatment of mild to moderate acne.

Willow Bark Extract

Anti-inflammatory plant extract with astringent properties.

Zinc Oxide

Anti-inflammatory, mineral-derived material that can be used to sooth irritation and form a protective barrier over irritated or damaged skin. Also possesses UV protection properties.

EXPERIMENTAL

This is the fun stuff! One of the most fascinating qualities of Korean skincare is the spirit of innovation and experimentation that permeates the culture when it comes to finding new, exciting, and beneficial skincare ingredients. Most of these ingredients are so new that they are still being studied for efficacy, but many of them do show early evidence of being able to perform functions such as brightening skin and accelerating wound healing. If the idea of trying something novel excites you, or if a little bit of whimsy with your skincare sounds like just what you need to stay true to your routine, these are the ingredients to look for!

Bee Venom

Anti-inflammatory and antibacterial properties. Expedites the healing of skin damage and inhibits acne-causing bacteria. The method for collecting the bee venom does not harm or kill the bees—in fact, some beekeepers say it actually increases the rate of honey production.

Bird's Nest

Made from nests built with the dried saliva of swiftlets. Rich in antioxidants, amino acids, and glycoprotein. Promotes healthy skin growth and stimulates skin's natural healing process.

Caviar / Salmon Egg

Rich in vitamins, minerals, proteins, amino acids, and lipids, with antioxidant and anti-inflammatory properties. Brightens skin, reduces redness, and promotes cell turnover.

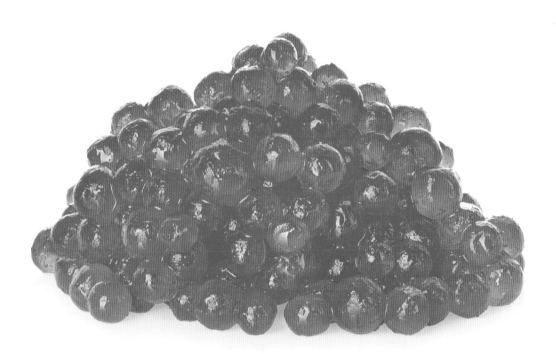

Cheese
Contains hydrating whey in addition to antioxidant vitamins A, B, and E.

Donkey Milk
Fatty acid and antioxidant rich with vitamins A, B, C, D, and E. Also contains proteins and ceramides. Provides moisturizing and anti-inflammatory effects.

Egg
Contains protein, lipid and some antioxidant content. Offers temporary skin-tightening effects.

Fermented Plants & Fruits
Includes any number or combination of fermented plants, flowers, or roots. The fermentation process often uses *lactobacillus*, a lactic acid probiotic, as a starter. Fermentation increases antioxidant concentrations and introduces new enzymes and amino acids. Effects on the skin can include hydration, brightening, soothing, redness reduction, and promotion of healthy skin growth.

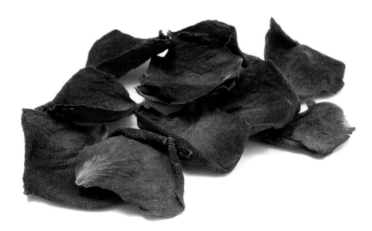

Goat Milk
Contains beneficial antioxidant vitamins A, B, and C as well as zinc, fatty acids, amino acids, and lactic acid. Provides moisture and soothing effects.

Horse Oil

Rendered horse fat with a similar fatty acid profile to human lipid composition. Easily absorbed, emollient properties as well as some anti-inflammatory effects.

Pearl

Amino acid-rich ingredient with anti-inflammatory and antimicrobial effects. Helps with collagen regeneration, redness reduction, spot lightening, and the treatment of acne.

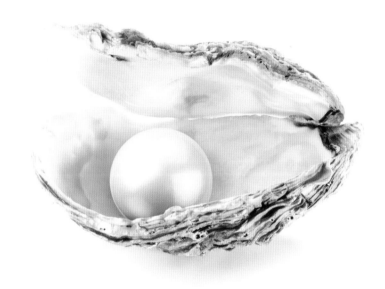

Pig Collagen

Skin-plumping, moisturizing humectant.

Placenta

Contains antioxidants and amino acids. Usually sheep-derived, but can occasionally be cow or even human-derived. Possesses moisturizing and temporary skin plumping abilities. Some unsubstantiated anti-aging claims are linked to the hormone content of this ingredient; there is also evidence that these hormones could be harmful, even when applied topically.

Snail Secretion Filtrate

Contains hyaluronic acid, glycoprotein enzymes, allantoin, glycolic acid, and copper peptides. Stimulates production of collagen and elastin, accelerates healing of wounded and damaged skin, and provides moisturizing benefits. Methods of collection for snail mucin do not harm or kill snails.

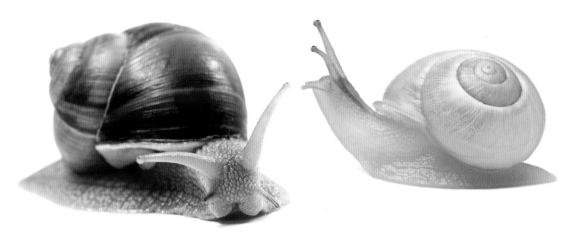

Starfish Extract

Potentially promotes the healing of wounded or damaged skin; may also provide some brightening and spot-lightening benefits.

Syn-ake

A synthetic form of snake venom which works by temporarily weakening facial muscle movements to prevent the formation or deepening of wrinkles.

Yeast (Saccharomyces) Ferment

An extract of live yeast cells with antioxidant and anti-inflammatory properties. Can help accelerate the healing of damaged skin, reduce redness, and provide hydrating benefits.

Yogurt

Fermented dairy ingredient with antioxidant and anti-inflammatory properties. Also contains lactic acid and zinc. Provides moisturizing, redness reduction, and brightening benefits. May also aid in the healing of acne.

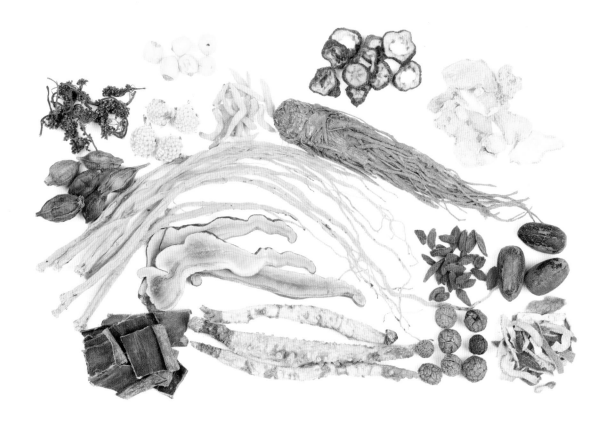

HANBANG

Hanbang is a popular term for Traditional Korean Medicine (TKM), which shares very similar origins, influences, and philosophies with Traditional Chinese Medicine (TCM). *Hangbang* ingredients are rooted in ancient tradition, though modern studies on the efficacy and function of the ingredients have been increasingly more common over the past few decades. These ingredients are herbal or sometimes animal-based, and are often fermented. *Hanbang* ingredients are especially popular in higher-end Korean skincare lines and products aimed at older woman looking for anti-aging alternatives. Interestingly, there is actually a bit of crossover between *hanbang* ingredients and what we now consider to be conventional skincare ingredients. In some instances, I actually had a difficult time deciding whether to classify a particular ingredient as Hanbang or conventional!

Asparagus Cochinchinensis Root (Wild Asparagus Root)

Possesses anti-inflammatory and antioxidant properties as well as amino acids. Promotes collagen synthesis and soothes irritation.

Astragalus Membranaceus Root (Astragalus Root)

Antioxidant root containing saponins and polysaccharides. Promotes the natural production of hyaluronic acid in the skin, stimulates collagen production, and contains an enzyme that helps lighten skin discolorations.

Centella Asiatica (Gotu Kola)

Antioxidant, antibacterial, and anti-inflammatory properties. Also possesses amino acids and some fatty acids. Hastens the healing of damaged skin, stimulates collagen production, and can reduce the severity of stretch mark and keloid scar appearance.

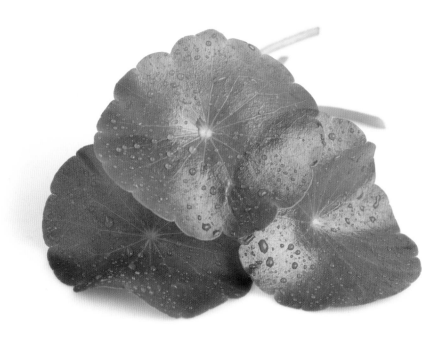

Chrysanthellum Indicum (Golden Chamomile)

Antioxidant and powerful anti-inflammatory herb that also displays antibacterial properties. Effective for redness reduction, especially in sensitive skin. Sometimes used as a treatment for mild rosacea.

Cnidium Officinale Root (Marsh Parsley)

Antibacterial, anti-fungal, and antioxidant-rich herb. Often used in anti-aging formulas for its free radical scavenging properties. Also sometimes included in products designed to treat skin rashes, such as eczema.

Cordyceps Sinensis (Caterpillar Mushroom)

Humectant and emollient skin conditioning herb with antioxidant properties.

Ginkgo Biloba (Maidenhair Tree)

Antibacterial, anti-fungal, antioxidant, and anti-inflammatory herb. Helpful for the treatment and prevention of acne, promotes blood circulation, and has also been shown to provide some supplementary protection against UV damage.

Lycium Chinense (Goji Berry)

Rich in amino acids, beta-carotene, vitamins B and C, as well as nicotinic acid. Helps stimulate collagen synthesis, and has been recently shown to have some brightening properties.

Nelumbo Nucifera (Lotus)

Anti-inflammatory and antioxidant plant with amino acids, fatty acids, as well as vitamin C and B. Stimulates blood circulation and the production of collagen. Also possesses hydrating, spot-lightening, and brightening abilities.

Panax Ginseng (Red, Fresh, White, and Wild Ginseng)

Powerful antioxidant and anti-inflammatory properties. Promotes healthy blood circulation, accelerates the healing of damaged skin, helps to stimulate collagen synthesis, and inhibits the formation of dark spots.

UV FILTERS

Utter the phrase "UV filter" to a photographer, and they'll assume you're referring to a camera accessory. Say "UV filter" to a skincare enthusiast, and they'll know you mean sunscreen! This section is dedicated to the ingredients found in Korean sunscreens and other multifunction sun-protection products (think BB creams) that either reflect harmful UVA and UVB rays away from our skin, or provide protection by absorbing and dissipating the rays to prevent UV damage.

UV filters can be a bit of a dry topic—they're definitely no party starters. But sun protection is hands-down the most effective way to prevent skin damage and premature aging. If it's not already the highest priority step in your daily skincare routine, it's time to put it on its much-deserved pedestal.

4-Methylbenzylidene Camphor

Protects against:
- UVB

Other names:
- 3-(4-Methylbenzylidene)bornan-2-one
- 3-(4-Methylbenzylidene)-dl-camphor
- Enzacamene

Amiloxate

Protects against:
- UVB

Other names:
- Isopentyl 4-methoxycinnamate
- Isoamyl p-methoxycinnamate

Avobenzone

Protects against:
- UVB
- UVA, though it degrades quickly in UVA light without the presence of a photostabilizer

Other names:

- 4-Tert-butyl-4-methoxydibenzoylmethane
- Butylmethoxydibenzoylmethane

Bemotrizinol

Protects against:

- UVB
- UVA

Other names:

- Anisotriazine
- Bis-ethylhexyloxyphenol methoxyphenyl triazine
- Escalol® S
- Tinosorb® S
- Tinosorb® S Aqua

Bisoctrizole

Protects against:

- UVB
- UVA

Other names:

- Tinosorb® M
- Milestab® 360

Diethylamino Hydroxybenzoyl Hexyl Benzoate

Protects against:

- UVA

Other names:

- Uvinul® A Plus

Ecamsule

Protects against:

- UVB
- UVA

Other names:

- Mexoryl® SX
- Terephthalylidene dicamphor sulfonic acid

Ethylhexyl Methoxycinnamate

Protects against:

- UVB

Other names:

- (E)-3-(4-methoxyphenyl) prop-2-enoic acid 2-ethylhexyl ester
- 2-Ethylhexyl-p-methoxycinnamate
- Eusolex® 2292
- Octinoxate
- Octyl methoxycinnamate
- Uvinul® MC80

Ethylhexyl Triazone

Protects against:

- UVB

Other names:

- Octyl triazone
- Uvinul® T 150

Octocrylene

Protects against:

- UVB
- UVA

Other names:

- Uvinul® N 539T

Octyl Salicylate

Protects against:
- UVB

Other names:
- 2-Ethylhexyl salicylate
- 2-Ethylhexyl ester salicylic acid
- 2-Ethylhexyl ester benzoic acid
- 2-hydroxy-2-ethylhexyl ester benzoic acid
- Ethyl hexyl salicylate
- Octisalate

Oxybenzone

Protects against:
- UVB
- UVA

Other names:
- 2-Hydroxy-4-methoxybenzophenone
- Benzophenone-3

Padimate O

Protects against:
- UVB

Other names:
- 2-Ethylhexyl dimethyl PABA
- Escalol® 507

Titanium Dioxide

Protects against:
- UVB
- UVA

Tris-Biphenyl Triazine

Protects against:
- UVB
- UVA

Other names:
- 2,4,6-Tris (p-biphenylyl)-s-triazine
- Tinosorb® A2B

Zinc Oxide

Protects against:
- UVB
- UVA

Other names:
- Z-Cote®

NEXT: PRODUCT CATEGORIES

Dr.G

BRIGHTENING UP
SUN

Mentor's Message

한층 더 밝아진 피부 톤 보정 선

| 피부 톤 보정 | 피지 조절 | 안티폴루션 콤플렉스 | 피부자극 테스트완료 |

OPENED DATE :   .   .

MY SKIN MENTOR Dr. G

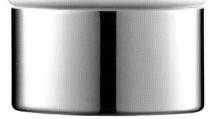

The sheer number of product types can be overwhelming and confusing to those new to the Korean skincare approach. If that's you, there's no need to be intimidated! In this section, we'll explore the vast array of product categories and their function. You'll find that using these products will become intuitive fairly quickly, and that for many of them, you may already be familiar with an equivalent or similar product in your existing routine. Furthermore, there's no pressure to incorporate every single product category into your routine! Once we move into building your routine, you'll see that you can incorporate as few or as many of these product types to accommodate your lifestyle, budget, and skincare goals.

POINT MAKEUP REMOVERS

This product is exactly what it sounds like—a makeup remover designed specifically for removing point makeup such as lipstick, eyeshadow, eyeliner, and mascara. Korean eye and lip makeup removers tend to be bi-phase formulas, which consist of a watery layer of liquid and an oil- or silicone-based liquid layer, that are designed to be shaken together before applying to a cotton pad for removing makeup.

The aspects of these removers I appreciate most are their affordability—even some the very inexpensive removers perform the same as higher-priced Western equivalents. I also appreciate their efficacy and their mildness. I am a very heavy-eyeliner wearer, and tend to lean on water-resistant eye makeup formulas, so having a remover that quickly and gently removes my eye makeup without a lot of tugging or unpleasant sensations is extremely important to me.

MAKEUP REMOVING CLEANSERS

Makeup removal is the first step in what's often referred to as the "double cleansing" process. Though double cleansing is common in many areas of the world, the concept also happens to be one of many defining characteristics of the Korean skincare approach. Double cleansing is a two-step cleansing process in which the first cleanser is designed to thoroughly remove makeup and sunscreen, and the second cleanser is designed to cleanse the skin of dirt, debris, residue, and in some cases, to exfoliate, once makeup has been removed.

Makeup removing cleansers are the first-step cleanser. An oil cleanser is the go-to standard for this step (and highly effective—it's a classic for a reason!), though sometimes micellar water, a cream cleanser, a multifunction cleanser, or a balm cleanser is used instead. Let's take a look at the different types of makeup removing cleansers typically found in the Korean skincare world.

OIL CLEANSERS

Oil cleansers are the most common choice for the first-step cleansing of a double-cleanse routine. These cleansers are oil based, but also contain emulsifying ingredients so they rinse away cleanly. Applied to dry skin, the oil breaks down makeup—even the waterproof stuff. Add a little water, and the cleanser turns into a milky lather that rinses away with no greasy residue.

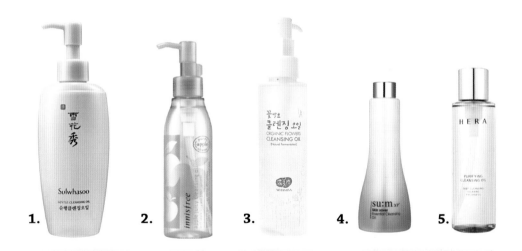

1. *Sulwhasoo Gentle Cleansing Oil* **/ 2.** *Innisfree Apple Juicy Cleansing Oil* **/ 3.** *Whamisa Organic Flower Cleansing Oil* **/ 4.** *Su:m37 Skin Saver Essential Cleansing Oil* **/ 5.** *Hera Purifying Cleansing Oil*

BALM CLEANSERS

Balm cleansers are a solid form of an oil cleanser. They have a soft, balmy texture that turns to oil as you rub it into your skin. It breaks down makeup just as an oil cleanser does, and transforms into milky, clean-rinsing lather when water is applied. You also have the option of tissuing this cleanser off in a pinch, but I highly recommend rinsing.

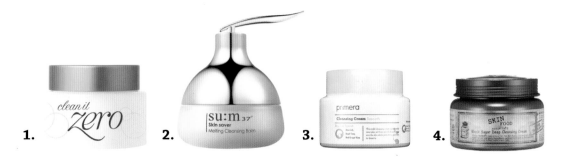

1. *Banila Co. Clean It Zero* / **2.** *Su:37 Skin Saver Melting Cleansing Balm* / **3.** *Primera Smooth Cleansing Cream* / **4.** *Skinfood Black Sugar Deep Cleansing Cream*

CREAM CLEANSERS

Cream cleansers are a fantastic choice for dry and sensitive skin, since they contain moisturizing ingredients and tend to have a slightly acidic pH. These cleansers have a thick, creamy consistency, not unlike a decadent moisturizer. They remove makeup beautifully when you massage them into dry skin. Add water and the cleanser will emulsify slightly, then rinse away clean. Like the balm cleanser, you can also tissue off this cleanser, but again, I recommend rinsing with water.

CLEANSING WATERS

If you're looking for a makeup-removing cleanser you don't have to rinse away, cleansing water—sometimes referred to as micellar water—is the way to go. Cleansing waters are composed of tiny clusters of surfactant molecules suspended in purified or spring water. Micellar waters have been big in France for a while now, and most skincare enthusiasts are familiar with the Bioderma or La Roche-Posay micellar products. Korean beauty brands have embraced the trend and elevated it by making an array of cleansing waters available, each with its own little twist. Some contain additional anti-inflammatory ingredients, while others contain antioxidants or skin calming extracts.

To use, just apply cleansing water to a clean cotton pad and wipe your makeup away. Because there's no need for rinsing, it's ideal for road trips and extended air travel.

MULTIFUNCTION CLEANSERS

Multifunction cleansers remove makeup and cleanse skin in a single step. They tend to have names that contain the phrase "all-in-one," "three-in-one," or "dual action." They usually start off as a viscous gel, then foam into a lather with water and rinse away, taking your dirt and makeup with it. They are generally effective in terms of removing makeup and dirt, though there's simply no substitute for a double cleanse.

Even though this cleanser is designed to reduce face washing, which in theory seems like it could be gentler on the skin, multifunction cleansers are often harsher and more stripping than other face cleansers, and can leave skin feeling tight and dry after washing. Most multifunction cleansers have a fairly high pH, so they aren't a great choice for those with sensitive or dehydrated skin. Someone with a strong moisture barrier and an urgent need to shave ninety seconds off of their cleansing routine may enjoy a multifunction cleanser.

FACIAL WIPES

Facial wipes are not a new concept, but the selections offered by Korean beauty brands tend to be gentler, less drying, and more luxurious than the wipes we're used to seeing. Sometimes people get apologetic about using facial wipes to remove makeup, but really—no need to apologize! Sometimes we're in a car, on a plane, or we're just exhausted, and a makeup removing wipe is exponentially better than not removing makeup at all.

FACIAL CLEANSERS

The goal of your second cleanse is to thoroughly remove any remaining dirt, oil, and residue that may be left behind on your face after you've removed your makeup. Second cleansers can take the form of a rich foam, a solid soap, or an exfoliating cleanser. Although there are many options available for this step, it's important to select a cleanser with a proper pH. Cleansers with a high pH can disrupt your skin's slightly acidic, protective barrier and raise your skin's pH over time, leaving it prone to acne, irritation, dehydration, and sensitivity. People with especially hardy moisture barriers may be able to tolerate a slightly higher pH than others.

Your face should never feel tight or dry after your second cleanse—it should feel clean, soft, and ready for the rest of your skincare ritual.

FOAMING CLEANSERS

Foaming cleansers are extremely seductive with their rich, voluminous lather and their soft, creamy consistency. They almost always smell like heaven. I once had a foaming cleanser that smelled and felt so wonderful that I actually daydreamed about going home and washing my face with it while I was at work. Unfortunately, many foaming cleansers—including the one I daydreamed about all day—have a very high pH (8.0–10.00), and are not great for long term use. The good news is, there are quite a few foaming cleansers available that have a great pH range; you just have to look for them. When choosing a foaming cleanser, the ideal pH range is between 5.0–6.0. People with oily skin that is not dehydrated or sensitive may be able to tolerate some of the higher pH foaming cleansers, but lower is still better as a general rule.

SOLID CLEANSERS

Solid cleansers are exactly what they sound like—cleansing bars and face soaps all fall into this category. I used to turn my nose up at all solid cleansers, thinking they weren't luxurious or gentle enough to use on my face. Most solid cleansers have a pH that's far too high for daily facial use. Soap, because of the way it's produced, is an alkaline product. But there are a few Korean brands that offer a class of solid cleansers that are moisturizing, luxurious, effective, and have either a neutral or slightly acidic pH that's ideal for the face. These solid cleansers are not true soaps, yet they produce a milky lather, and are very effective at removing dirt while being gentle and non-drying on the skin. My favorite solid cleansers are so effective that they can actually be used to remove makeup for my first cleanse as well, making them ideal for travel. I'm finding that many of them are more luxurious than my favorite foaming cleansers were!

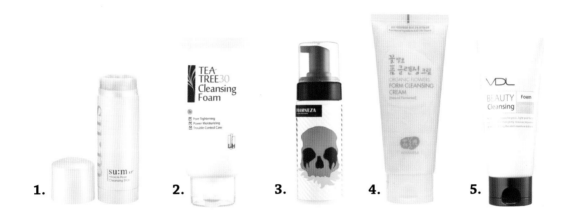

1. *Su:m37 Miracle Rose Cleansing Stick* / **2.** *Leejiham (LJH) Tea Tree 30 Cleansing Foam* / **3.***Too Cool For School Foamneza Foaming Cleanser* / **4.** *Whamisa Organic Flowers Foam Cleansing Cream* / **5.** *VDL Beauty Cleansing Foam (Sensitive)*

EXFOLIATING CLEANSERS

Exfoliating cleansers remove dead skin cells to reveal a brighter, smoother complexion. They also help with reducing the appearance of pore size as well as preventing blackheads. Some exfoliating cleansers are manual exfoliators, meaning they contain sugar or cellulose granules that physically remove the dead skin, while others use acids or enzymes to break down the bonds that adhere dead skin cells to newer cells. Manual exfoliators tend to have the word "polish" or "scrub" in the product name, while chemical exfoliators use words such as "peeling" or "enzyme." They can come in a range of forms including gel, powder, or a foaming liquid. They're not intended for daily use; two–three times a week is frequent enough to keep your complexion bright and fresh, but not so frequent that you risk over exfoliating and damaging your skin.

TONERS / SKIN / BOOSTERS

We've all heard of a facial toner, but it's important to know that a typical Korean toner is vastly different in terms of function and ingredients from a Western-style toner. Western toners are designed to provide an additional cleansing function and tend to have astringent properties. A Korean toner, sometimes referred to as a "skin" or "booster," is designed to add moisture to the skin that might be stripped away during the cleansing process, and to increase the penetration of the skincare products that follow.

Some brands have separate toners and boosters, in which case the booster is applied first to prepare the skin for more products, followed by the toner, which is designed to soften the skin. However, in many skincare lines, the toner and booster are the same product.

Although most Korean toners are of the hydrating variety, there are exceptions. There are a handful of brands that offer low pH, AHA- or BHA-based toners, which provide light exfoliation and adjust the skin's pH after cleansing. Many people who use an acid-based toner will also follow up with a hydrating toner or booster.

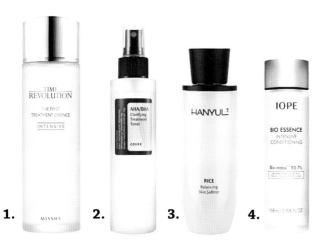

1. *Missha Time Revolution: The First Treatment Essence Intensive* **/ 2.** *COSRX AHA/BHA Clarifying Treatment Toner* **/ 3.** *Hanyul Rice Balancing Skin Softner* **/ 4.** *Iope Bio-Essence Intensive Conditioning*

ESSENCES / SERUMS / AMPOULES

An essence is a lightly hydrating liquid containing skin-beneficial ingredients, usually targeted toward specific skin concerns such as hyperpigmentation, dullness, aging, or acne. Its texture can range from that of a watery toner to a thicker, more serum-like consistency. Though an essence and a serum can often be very similar, serums generally have a higher concentration of beneficial ingredients. An ampoule is used to describe a product that's more densely concentrated than a serum, but sometimes the terms "serum" and "ampoule" are used interchangeably.

It's not uncommon to have an essence, serum, and an ampoule in a routine, or more than one of any one of the individual product types, in order to target multiple skin troubles.

5. *Hanyul White Chrysanthemum Powder Serum* **/ 6.** *C20 Pure Viramin C21.5 Advanced Serum* **/ 7.** *Leejiham Tea Tree 90 Essence* **/ 8.** *Missha Time Revolution: Night Repair Science Activator Borabit Ampoule*

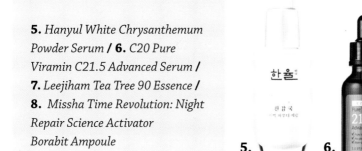

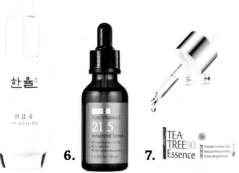

EMULSIONS

An emulsion, sometimes referred to as a lotion, is a moisturizing treatment. It is lighter than a cream, but designed to hydrate and moisturize skin, and contains many of the same active and beneficial ingredients found in an essence, though it's generally less concentrated.

For people with oily skin or who live in a humid climate, this might be the only moisturizer in their skincare routine. Those with dry skin types may opt to apply a more occlusive cream over the emulsion, particularly in the evening.

FACE OILS

Face oils have gained a lot of popularity in the Korean beauty landscape, just as they have across the Americas in recent years. The difference is that Korean brands tend to offer oil blends designed for specific skin concerns. These oils are combined with complimentary ingredients that help increase absorbency and further treat skin concerns. For many, the essence step is where a face oil would typically fit into a Korean skincare routine, although many prefer to use a face oil in place of the emulsion step.

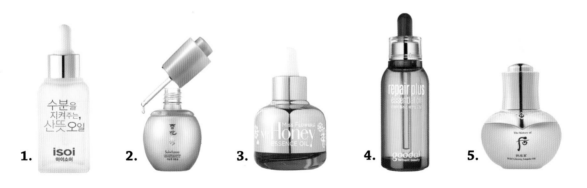

1. Isoi Moisture Face Oil / 2. Sulwhasoo Concentrated Ginseng Renewing Essential Oil / 3. Banila Co. Miss Flower & Mr. Honey Essence Oil / 4. Goodal Repair Plus Essential Oil / 5. The History of Whoo Wild Ginseng AmpouleOil

MOISTURIZING CREAMS

Creams are meant to provide moisture. For some people, especially those with dry skin, they are an extra moisturizing step in addition to an emulsion or face oil. They are generally thicker than emulsions, often have occlusive properties, and usually come packaged in a jar rather than a pump bottle or tube. Many people skip this step, particularly those with oily skin or people who live in more humid climates, opting to use an emulsion or face oil as their only moisturizer. Those of us with mature or dry skin will find this step indispensable!

However, it's important to note that not all moisturizing creams are heavy or occlusive. In fact, one of the great advantages Korean skincare brings to people with oily skin types is the vast number of products that cater to them. There is a huge array of moisturizing creams that are composed primarily of humectant ingredients, which provide hydration without being heavy or smothering.

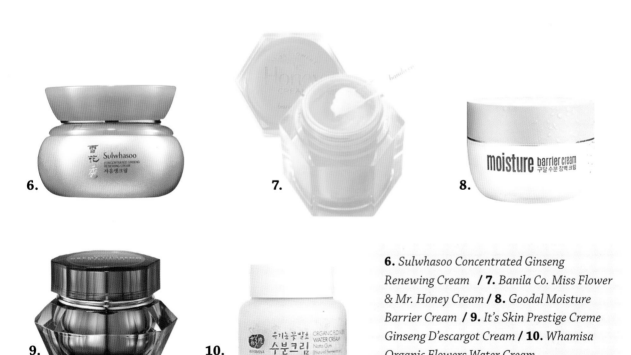

6. *Sulwhasoo Concentrated Ginseng Renewing Cream* **/ 7.** *Banila Co. Miss Flower & Mr. Honey Cream* **/ 8.** *Goodal Moisture Barrier Cream* **/ 9.** *It's Skin Prestige Creme Ginseng D'escargot Cream* **/ 10.** *Whamisa Organic Flowers Water Cream*

EYE CREAMS

If you're an eye cream fan, you'll be happy to know that there is a vast selection of Korean eye creams available. Eye creams aren't a necessary step for many—your regular facial products should perform just as well in your eye area as they do on the rest of your face. However, there are cases where having a separate eye cream is extremely beneficial. You should consider a product specifically made for your eye area if:

- The skin in your eye area has a significantly different moisturizing need than the rest of your face.
- The skin around your eyes tends to be drier than the rest of your face, then it makes sense to use a richer cream in that area. Conversely, if your facial cream is too rich for your eye area or you're experiencing milia seeds from your regular facial moisturizer, it's smart to use a lighter cream or gel for your eyes.
- You're not ready for an anti-aging ingredient such as retinol on your face, but your eyes are in need of some extra wrinkle-fighting power.
- You want to treat an issue that you have only around your eyes, such as dullness, darkness, or puffiness.

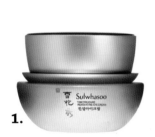 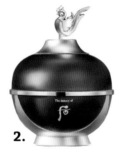 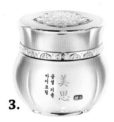 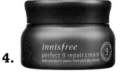

1. *Sulwhasoo Timetreasure Renovating Eye Cream* **/ 2.** *The History of Whoo Hwanyu Eye Cream* **/**
3. *Missha MISA Geumsul Vitalizing Eye Cream* **/ 4.** *Innisfree Perfect 9 Repair Eye Cream*

SPOT TREATMENTS

A spot treatment can be a number of things—acne treatment, whitening serum, wrinkle filler, etc. Many acne treatments fall into this category. There are spot treatments for other skin concerns as well, such as lighteners that contain ingredients designed to fade stubborn hyperpigmentation spots, and there are even spot treatments that address the appearance of lines and wrinkles.

The qualities that define a spot treatment can be a bit nebulous, but some good qualifiers include:

- The product does not clearly fall into any other product categories
- The product is extremely focused on a single skincare concern
- The product is highly concentrated
- It comes in a ridiculously tiny tube or jar

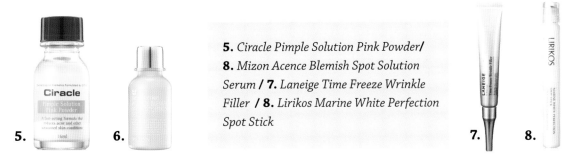

5. *Ciracle Pimple Solution Pink Powder/* **8.** *Mizon Acence Blemish Spot Solution Serum* / **7.** *Laneige Time Freeze Wrinkle Filler* / **8.** *Lirikos Marine White Perfection Spot Stick*

5.   **6.**   **7.**   **8.**

SUNSCREEN

Sun protection is simply the most effective, repeatedly proven defense we have against dark spots, skin damage, fine lines, and wrinkles. I can't emphasize enough how essential a stand-alone sunscreen is when it comes to keeping skin healthy and in slowing the effects of aging! I specify "stand-alone" for a reason. Many people use a daytime moisturizer or foundation with built-in sun protection, but the unfortunate truth is that those products are not supplying anyone with adequate UV protection. The reason for this is that we need to use ¼ teaspoon of sunscreen on our face in order to obtain the amount of sun protection advertised on the product label—¼ teaspoon is a lot! It's about the diameter of a cherry—and most people aren't using that much moisturizer or (we can hope) foundation.

The good news is that Korean skincare brands offer a wide variety of amazing stand-alone sunscreen formulas. Forget about the thick, white, pasty sunblocks you slather on for a day at the beach—Korean sunscreen formulas feel weightless, absorb quickly, and wear extremely well underneath makeup.

When choosing a Korean sunscreen, look for a formula that offers a high SPF (that's the UVB protection) and a high PA rating (that's the UVA protection). The PA rating is a measurement of UVA protection, used for any sunscreen manufactured and sold in Asian countries. The PA rating system originated in Japan, and is based on the widely used PPD (Persistent Pigment Darkening) method, a system of measuring UVA protection used in European countries.

The PA system ranges from PA+ to PA++++, and each level corresponds with a range of PPD measurements. Here's how the PA system equates with the PPD system:

- PA+ = 2–3 PPD
- PA++ = 4–7 PPD
- PA+++ = 8–5 PPD
- PA++++ = 16+ PPD

Note: *As of 2015, Korean sunscreens only go up to PA+++, as the PA++++ criterion was newly introduced in Japan at the end of 2012 and has not yet expanded out of the country.*

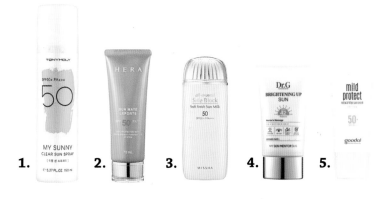

1. TonyMoly My Sunny Clear Sun Spray SPF50 PA+++ / 2. Hera Sun Mate Leports SPF50 PA+++ / 3. Missha All-Around Safe Block Soft Finish Sun Milk SPF50 PA+++ / 4. Dr.G Brightening Up Sun Cream SPF42 PA+++ / 5. Goodal Mild Protect Natural Filter Sun Cream SPF50 PA+++

SHEET MASKS

Sheet masks are thin sheets of material soaked in a treatment essence or serum designed to infuse the skin with an immediate burst of hydration, and they may also target specific skin concerns. They're applied to the face, and have holes cut out for the eyes, nose, and mouth. Sheet masks can do a number of things—some of them are moisturizing, some are exfoliating, some are brightening, and some are nourishing. They also possess the unfailing ability to make anyone look like an axe murderer for the fifteen to twenty minute duration they're being worn, but I consider this a selling point. Most sheet masks are meant to be applied after the toner/booster step, and for some people, they replace the essence/serum step altogether.

The essences the sheet masks are soaked in are truly what make or break a particular mask. All sheet masks contain a plentiful helping of humectants, which is why the hydrating effects tend to be so instant and dramatic. The most popular humectants used in sheet mask essences are glycerin, butylene glycol, and propylene glycol, though some of the nicer masks may use hyaluronic acid, honey, or aloe. In addition to the humectant ingredients, the essences also contain penetration enhancers to help the skin absorb the product, as well as additional ingredients designed to target specific skin conditions. Popular skin-beneficial ingredients include niacinamide, green tea, ginseng, and snail secretion filtrate, but in the world of sheet masks, anything is possible.

Sheet masks are available in a few different materials, and each of the varying materials performs a little differently.

FIBER/PULP

Fiber masks and pulp masks are the most prevalent sheet masks. They're typically one continuous piece of material and made from cotton, paper, or some kind of synthetic cellulose. These types of sheet masks are abundantly available, come in an endless array of "flavors," and generally do an effective job replenishing hydration levels in the skin, provided the essence they're soaking in is plentiful and formulated well.

HYDRO GEL

Hydro gels are quickly gaining popularity in the sheet mask scene. These sheet masks usually come in two parts—one for the top half of the face and another for the bottom half. The warmth of your skin helps the mask adhere closely to the contours of your face, making for a close fit, though sliding is still often an issue.

The hydro gel mask is not soaked in essence; instead, the essence is actually mixed in with the gelatin during production. For this reason, evaporation isn't much of a problem. These masks feel extremely cool and soothing during wear. Hydro gel masks are generally priced a bit higher than fiber and pulp masks.

BIO CELLULOSE

Bio cellulose masks are the latest material to burst onto the sheet mask scene. Bio cellulose is a material used in biomedicine as artificial skin to heal burns and treat wounds, and is now being utilized by the cosmetic industry. What makes it a unique material is its ability to hold 100 times its dry weight in fluid, which is a great quality for a product designed to hold essence against the skin for an extended period of time. These masks are made of a single sheet, which adheres closely and evenly to the skin. Additionally, the material is 100 percent biodegradable. Bio cellulose sheet masks are priced similarly to hydro gels.

1. 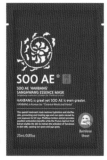 **2.** 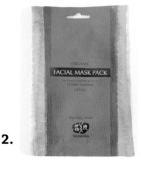 **3.**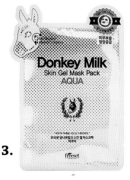

1. *Soo Ae Hanbang Sanghwang Essence Mask* **/ 2.** *Whamisa Organic Sea Kelp Facial Sheet Mask* **/ 3.** *Freeset Donkey Milk Skin Gel Mask Pack Aqua*

SLEEPING PACKS

A sleeping pack, also called a sleeping mask, is an overnight skin treatment that comes in a tub or a tube. It's designed to be applied on the face as your last skincare step in the evening in order to provide hydration and other skincare benefits while you sleep. It can be used in addition to or in lieu of a nighttime moisturizing cream, depending on your needs.

The frequency of use varies depending on your preferences—some people find it beneficial to use a sleeping pack every night, while others only reach for it a few times a week. If you're a side sleeper and worried about covering your pillow in greasy face products—don't be. Most sleeping packs absorb completely in the same way a moisturizer does. Additionally, there are so many different textures, thicknesses, and absorbency rates in sleeping pack products, if you're not happy with the first one you try, it's worth it to keep experimenting. There's bound to be an option that you'll fall in love with.

4. 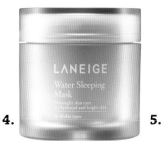 **5.** 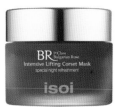 **6.** 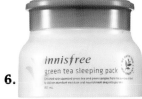 **7.**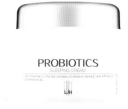

4. *Laneige Water Sleeping Mask* **/ 5.** *Isoi Bulgarian Rose Intensive Lifting Corest Mask* **/ 6.** *Innisfree Green Tea Sleeping Pack* **/ 7.** *Leejuham (LJH) Probiotics Sleeping Cream*

SKIN FINISHER

Skin finishers are a relatively new category of product in the skincare world, and their function blurs the line a bit between skincare and makeup. They are light in texture, and usually have some sort of opalescent quality imparted by the micronized pearl particles they contain. As a skincare product, skin finishers contain ingredients that help form a thin barrier over your other products, helping to maintain moisture throughout the day and maximize their skincare benefits. Skin finisher formulas also tend to include plant extracts with antioxidant, anti-inflammatory, or other skin-benefiting properties. As a makeup product, the micronized pearl has a luminizing effect on the skin, and the finisher also acts as a primer to help keep your makeup in place throughout the day.

WASH-OFF MASKS

Wash-off masks are another item that you're probably already familiar with. If you're a fan of these types of treatments, you'll be excited to learn that there's a huge range of spectacular products in this category offered by Korean beauty brands! They vary in both texture and function, ranging from simple moisturizing masks, to exfoliating treatments, to brightening masks. The application method is the same as the one you already know: apply the mask treatment to clean skin, leave it on for the period of time specified on the packaging, then rinse away, and continue the rest of your skincare routine.

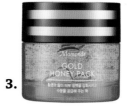

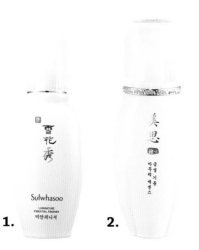

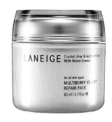

1. Sulwhasoo Luminature Essential Finisher / 2. Missha Geumsul Giyun Vitalizing Finisher / 3. Mamonde Gold Honey Pack / 4. Laneige Multiberry Yogurt Pack

1.   2.   3.   4.

MASSAGE CREAM

A massage cream, sometimes called a massage mask or massage pack, is a rich cream or balm that provides an intensive moisturizing treatment for the face. This product is designed for people who are suffering from fatigued, lackluster, or dull skin. They are massaged generously but gently onto clean skin for anywhere from two to five minutes. Methods for removal vary widely depending on the product: some products are to be tissued off, some rinse with water, and others are not to be removed at all, but are simply pressed into the skin. One thing all massage packs do have in common is that they are all very decadent, and they are an especially luxurious treat for dry skin.

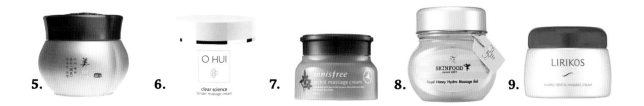

5. *Missha MISA Yei Hyun Glowing Massage* **/ 6.** *O Hui Clear Science Tender Massage Cream* **/ 7.** *Innisfree Orchid Massage Cream* **/ 8.** *Skinfood Royal Honey Hydro Massage Gel* **/ 9.** *Lirikos Marine Revital Massage Cream*

FACIAL MISTS

Facial mists are watery sprays fortified with plant extracts and hydrating ingredients. They come in bottles or cans, and are meant to be used as a supplemental hydrator throughout the day. They're very useful in both warm and cold weather. On hot summer days, they're a refreshing burst of cool relief after spending time in the sun. In cold weather, they offer hydration after spending time in the dry air caused by central heating systems. The formulas for facial mists are light, watery, and non-greasy, which makes them compatible with all skin types, and they are light enough that they can be sprayed over makeup.

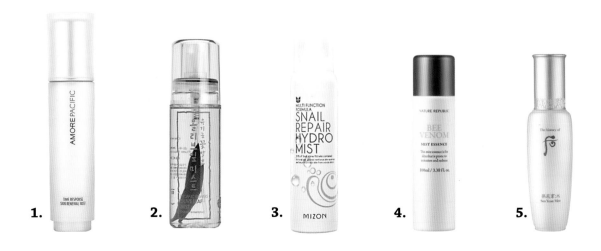

1. *Amorepacific Time Response Skin Renewal Mist* **/ 2.** *Whamisa Organic Flowers Olive Leaf Mist* **/**
3. *Mizon Snail Repair Hydro Mist* **/ 4.** *Nature Republic Bee Venom Mist Essence* **/ 5.** *The History of Whoo Soo Yeon Mist*

UP NEXT: BUILDING A ROUTINE

Building your customized Korean skincare routine shouldn't be intimidating—it should be fun! Once you know what you're looking for and what you want to avoid, the process is very enjoyable. The best way to start building your routine is by assessing your skin type and identifying your skincare concerns. If you have a clear idea of what your skincare goals are, you'll cut out a lot of guesswork when it comes to selecting products that will help you achieve your best complexion.

Additionally, it's important to keep in mind that everyone's skin is different. People may have different ingredient sensitivities, and there may be outside factors that impact the efficacy of certain skincare products such as climate, air quality, or lifestyle differences. As you build your routine and introduce new products, pay close attention to how your skin looks and feels. Even if a product is highly praised and well-loved by many, there's always a chance it might not be right for you.

Your routine should be customized for your needs and lifestyle. The most effective skincare routine is a consistent routine, so if an elaborate eight- to twelve-step skincare routine doesn't sound like something that fits your lifestyle, don't worry! You can create an effective routine with just a handful of the right products. On the other hand, if you have the discipline, desire, and the need for a more elaborate routine, you'll be able to find products that address all of your skin concerns.

INTRODUCING NEW PRODUCTS

PATCH TESTING

When trying any new skincare product, there's always a risk that you could react negatively to an ingredient. To prevent a full-blown catastrophe, be sure to patch test new products before you incorporate them into your routine. To test, apply the new product to your test area, and watch it over the next twenty-four to forty-eight hours to see how your skin reacts. The best places to test are behind your ear or on the underside of your forearm.

Some people will react fairly immediately to a product, while others take a bit longer to show negative effects. With so many variables at play, it's wise to patch test for at least a couple of days before committing a product to your entire face.

ONE PRODUCT AT A TIME

It's also best to introduce only one new product at a time. If you introduce multiple new products at once and have a bad reaction, you'll have no way of knowing which product is the culprit! Try to space your new product introductions apart by at least a week.

COMMON QUESTIONS

Do all my products need to be from the same skincare line?

They can be, but they don't have to be. If you're just beginning your Korean skincare journey, using a single line can be an easy and straightforward way to familiarize yourself with the steps in your new routine. Using the same line for all your products is also a safe choice because the formulations have been designed to work well with one another, and can be especially beneficial if you've chosen a line to address a single skin concern, such as evening your skin tone. All of the products in that line will contain ingredients that address that particular issue, and work in synergy with one another.

However, if you have multiple skin issues you'd like to address, your best solutions won't all come from the same skincare line. Unless you have very few skin concerns, you'll need to shop different lines to assemble an optimal routine for your skincare goals. Also, as you progress in your skincare journey, you're going to find a variety of product formulations that work really well for you, and chances are they will not only be from separate lines, but different brands as well. Assembling a routine composed of all the "best in show" products for your skin is incredibly effective and satisfying, but it will be nearly impossible to make that happen if you restrict yourself to a single skincare line indefinitely.

How long will it take to know if a product is effective?

Your facial skin renews itself over the course of a month. You might be able to see some of the more basic effects a product has on your skin within a couple of days, such as the amount of moisture it provides or whether there are any short term brightening, soothing, or anti-inflammatory improvements. But you won't be able to get a solid idea of what a product's long term impact will be until about four weeks into its usage.

The exception, of course, is if you have a bad reaction to a product, such as irritation, contact dermatitis—really, anything negative that happens suddenly after starting a new product. If this happens, you should stop using that product immediately.

Is it possible to use too many products?

It is! And you'll know when you've overdone it. Pay attention to how your face looks and feels, especially when you're working on assembling a new skincare routine. If your face is consistently too sticky, too oily, too dry, too *anything*—you're probably using too many products, or too much of one particular thing. The exception to this rule is if you find your skin is suddenly too perfect. In that case, everything is fine and you should carry on with what you're doing.

LAYERING & ORDER OF APPLICATION

When beginning a Korean skincare routine for the first time, figuring out the order in which products should be applied can be overwhelming. In this section, we'll be exploring some basic guidelines to help steer you through your product application. Here are some core general guidelines for determining the order of your application:

1. Apply your products in order from the lightest weight to the heaviest. This allows for maximum absorption of each of the products, and ensures that your thinner, water-rich layers are safely tucked beneath your smoothing emollient and occlusive products.

2. Sometimes brands will prescribe a product order that deviates slightly from the lightest-to-heaviest approach. In this instance, it's best to follow the brand's recommendations.

3. If you're using a pH-dependent product such as a low-pH acid toner, an AHA, BHA, or a vitamin C serum, it's best to apply those at the beginning of your routine, just after cleansing. These products function best when skin is at its natural, slightly acidic pH, and applying other products first could interfere with their performance.

The following are examples of application order for morning and evening routines. Your own routine may differ, but these provide a good starting point for determining the sequence of your regemin.

Morning Routine Layering Examples

SIMPLE

STEP 1: CLEANSE

STEP 2: HYDRATING TONER

STEP 3: ESSENCE

STEP 4: EMULSION or OIL

STEP 5: SUNSCREEN

INTERMEDIATE

STEP 1: CLEANSE

STEP 2: HYDRATING TONER

STEP 3: ESSENCE

STEP 4: SERUM

STEP 5: EMULSION or OIL

STEP 6: SUNSCREEN

ADVANCED
NORMAL / DRY

STEP 1: CLEANSE

STEP 2: LOW PH TONER

STEP 3: VITAMIN C*

STEP 4: HYDRATING TONER

STEP 5: ESSENCE

STEP 6: EMULSION or FACE OIL

STEP 7: CREAM

STEP 8: SUNSCREEN

ADVANCED
OILY / COMBINATION

STEP 1: CLEANSE

STEP 2: LOW PH TONER

STEP 3: BHA SERUM*

STEP 4: VITAMIN C*

STEP 5: HYDRATING TONER

STEP 6: ESSENCE

STEP 7: EMULSION or OIL

STEP 8: SUNSCREEN

Optional wait time of ten to fifteen minutes for pH-dependent products to maximize efficacy. If using both vitamin C and BHA, you can apply both before beginning your wait time. Always wear daytime sunscreen when using pH-dependent products!

Evening Routine Layering Examples

SIMPLE

STEP 1: MAKEUP REMOVAL CLEANSE

STEP 2: FACIAL CLEANSE

STEP 3: HYDRATING TONER

STEP 4: ESSENCE

STEP 5: EMULSION or OIL

INTERMEDIATE

STEP 1: MAKEUP REMOVAL CLEANSE

STEP 2: FACIAL CLEANSE

STEP 3: HYDRATING TONER

STEP 4: SHEET MASK

STEP 5: SERUM

STEP 6: EMULSION or OIL

STEP 7: SLEEPING PACK

ADVANCED
NORMAL / DRY

STEP 1: MAKEUP REMOVAL CLEANSE

STEP 2: FACIAL CLEANSE

STEP 3: LOW PH TONER

STEP 4: AHA or BHA SERUM*

STEP 5: HYDRATING TONER

STEP 6: SHEET MASK

STEP 7: AMPOULE / SERUM

STEP 8: CREAM

STEP 9: SLEEPING PACK

STEP 10: SPOT TREATMENT

ADVANCED
OILY / COMBINATION

STEP 1: MAKEUP REMOVAL CLEANSE

STEP 2: FACIAL CLEANSE

STEP 3: LOW PH TONER

STEP 4: AHA or BHA SERUM*

STEP 5: HYDRATING TONER

STEP 6: SHEET MASK

STEP 7: AMPOULE / SERUM

STEP 8: EMULSION or OIL

STEP 9: SLEEPING PACK

STEP 10: SPOT TREATMENT

Optional wait time of ten to fifteen minutes for pH-dependent products to maximize efficacy. If using both AHA and BHA, you can apply both before beginning your wait time.

SKINCARE PRODUCT SHOPPING CHEAT SHEETS

The most important part of product selection is in choosing products that address your skincare goals. Whether you're shopping online or in-person, it can be helpful to have a quick reference of what you're looking for to help you determine how effective a product will be for your need. In the pages that follow, you'll find a series of cheat sheets for various skin types and concerns. Use these as a reference as you shop for your new Korean skincare products, and let the fun begin!

BY SKIN TYPE

GOALS:	What you should be aiming for
PRODUCTS:	Which product types will help you get there
AVOID:	What will hinder your progress
KEYWORDS:	Words to look for in product names and descriptions

Normal Skin

GOALS: Keeping your skin healthy and slowing the onset of aging by maintaining hydration levels, loading up with antioxidants, and protecting yourself against UV damage.

PRODUCTS: Refreshing hydrating toners and first essences, antioxidant-rich serums or ampoules, light emulsions or face oils.

AVOID: Products designed for skin concerns you don't have. When in doubt, products made for combination skin are usually a good choice for those with normal skin as well.

KEYWORDS: Combination, balancing, nutrition, aqua, hydrating

Dry Skin

GOALS: Dry skin loves humectants, so layer them on, then seal them in with a veil of occlusive or emollient moisture. It's okay to be indulgent! Dry skin is one of the best skin types to have if you enjoy a decadent skincare routine.

PRODUCTS: Humectant-rich hydrating toners, face oils, emulsions, and moisturizing creams with emollient and occlusive properties.

AVOID: Alkaline/high-pH cleansers and products made for oily skin. These products are easy to spot, and usually contain the words pore, sebum, oil-free, or tightening

KEYWORDS: Aqua, bomb (e.g., water bomb), nutrition, rejuvenate, rich, moisture

Oily Skin

GOALS: Hydration is extremely important, but some heavier products can make oily skin worse. Focus on primarily humectent moisturizers so your face will stay hydrated without feeling greasy.

PRODUCTS: Refreshing, hydrating toners, light emulsions, and gel-based creams. Pore serums and clay or charcoal-based masks are also great choices.

AVOID: Heavier face oils and richer, more occlusive creams

KEYWORDS: Balancing, oil-free, pore

Combination Skin

GOALS: Humectants to the rescue again—they provide beneficial moisture to all skin types. Seal in the humectant moisture with an emollient face oil or emulsion on the dry areas of your face.

PRODUCTS: Refreshing, hydrating toners and first essences, antioxidant-rich serums or ampoules, light emulsions or face oils

AVOID: Products that are either far too occlusive for your oily areas or not moisturizing enough for dry areas. If your dry and oily zones areas are very different, it's okay to use different products for parts of your face.

KEYWORDS: Combination, balancing, aqua, and hydrating

BY SKIN CONCERN

TIPS: Hints for approaching your concern

INGREDIENTS: Which ingredients will help address skin concerns

KEYWORDS: Words to look for in product names and descriptions

Acne

TIPS:	Using an entire line of anti-acne products can be harsh on the skin. Start with an essence or serum designed for acne while keeping the rest of your routine optimized for other skin concerns.

INGREDIENTS

TREAT & PREVENT ACTIVE ACNE:	Azealic acid, bee venom, betaine salicylate, charcoal, clay, ginkgo biloba, glycolic acid, l-ascorbic acid, lactic acid, malic acid, niacinamide, retinoids, tea tree oil
SOOTHE INFLAMMATION & REDNESS:	Adenosine, aloe vera, bee venom, donkey milk, ginkgo biloba, honey, nelumbo nucifera, propolis, snail secretion filtrate, willow bark extract, yogurt, zinc oxide
TREAT & PREVENT MARKS AND SCARS:	Arbutin, astragalus membranaceus root, azealic acid, betaine salicylate, centella asiatica, chrysanthellum indicum, glycolic acid, l-ascorbic acid, lactic acid, malic acid, licorice root, morus alba/ mulberry extract, nelumbo nucifera, niacinamide, snail secretion filtrate, retinoids
KEYWORDS:	Trouble, blemish, pore, clear, BHA, spot, tea tree

Dullness, Hyperpigmentation, & Uneven Tone

TIPS:
Before investing in an entire routine focused on only perfecting skin tone or on brightening dullness, try a single essence, serum, or ampoule geared toward that concern. You may find that one product does the trick, allowing you to focus on other concerns for remaining products in your lineup.

INGREDIENTS:
Arbutin, astragalus membranaceus root, azealic acid, betaine salicylate, centella asiatica, chrysanthellum indicum, glycolic acid, l-ascorbic acid, lactic acid, malic acid, licorice root, morus alba/mulberry extract, nelumbo nucifera, niacinamide, snail secretion filtrate, retinoids

KEYWORDS:
Bright, white, mela, snow

Dehydration

TIPS:
Dehydration is the result of a damaged moisture barrier. The best way to repair and strengthen your skin's protective barrier is to keep it well-moisturized with humectants sealed beneath a layer of emollient and occlusive products rich in fatty acids. It's especially important for dehydrated skin to cleanse with products that have a lower pH of 5.0—6.0.

INGREDIENTS:
Aloe vera, animal-based oils, ceramide, cocoa butter, donkey milk, goat milk, honey, lactobacillus, mango seed butter, plant-based carrier oils (e.g., argan, olive, sesame, etc.), shea butter, squalane

KEYWORDS:
Nutrition, healing, repair, rich, EX

Wrinkles & Fine Lines

TIPS:
There is a very short list of ingredients that can actually reduce wrinkles long term. To delay the onset of future lines, wear sunscreen daily, keep skin hydrated, and nourish your skin with antioxidants.

INGREDIENTS

REDUCE EXISTING FINE LINES & WRINKLES:
Azealic acid, glycolic acid, I-ascorbic acid, lactic acid, malic acid, niacinamide, retinoids

PREVENT FINE LINES & WRINKLES:
All moisturizing ingredients, all UV filters, niacinamide, retinoids, antioxidant extracts

TEMPORARILY REDUCE WRINKLE APPEARANCE:
Caffiene, collagen, glycerin, hyaluronic acid, syn-ake

KEYWORDS:
Anti-aging, defense, future, lifting, refine, renew, renovate, repair, rejuvenate

Sensitivity

TIPS:
No two sensitive skins are alike. Your individual sensitives to specific ingredients or environmental conditions will differ greatly from someone else's, even if their symptoms are similar to yours.

INGREDIENTS:
Aloe vera, (betaine, ceramide, chamomile, chrysanthellum indicum, cnidium officinale, cocoa butter, cucumber, donkey milk, goat milk, green tea, honey, lactobacillus, mango seed butter, oatmeal, plant-based carrier oils (e.g., argan, olive, sesame, etc.), propolis, shea butter, squalane, willow bark extract, yeast (sacchromyces) ferment

KEYWORDS:
Sensitive, gentle, calming, soothing

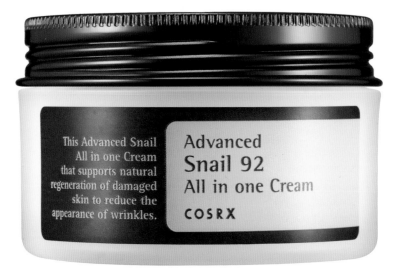

To show you how different routines can be from person to person, we've rounded up our favorite K-beauty bloggers, all with varying skin types and concerns, to share their skincare routines with you! We've also included our own routines. Whether you're looking for a starting point, or you're seeking out some inspiring ways to change your current skincare lineup, these examples may have just what you need to take your skin to the next level.

Remember that everyone's skin is unique, so people have varying sensitivities and levels of responsiveness to product formulations and ingredients. Even if your concerns are identical to someone else's, there's always a possibility that a product that worked miracles for them won't be as magical for you. Don't forget to patch test, introduce one new product at a time, and don't be afraid to do a little research before splurging on something new!

This section includes example skincare routines from:

FANSERVICED-B

RYANRAROAR

SNOW WHITE & THE ASIAN PEAR

FIFTY SHADES OF SNAIL

HELLO PRETTY BIRD!

MEMORABLE DAYS

THE WANDERLUST PROJECT

THE BEAUTY WOLF

SKIN & TONICS

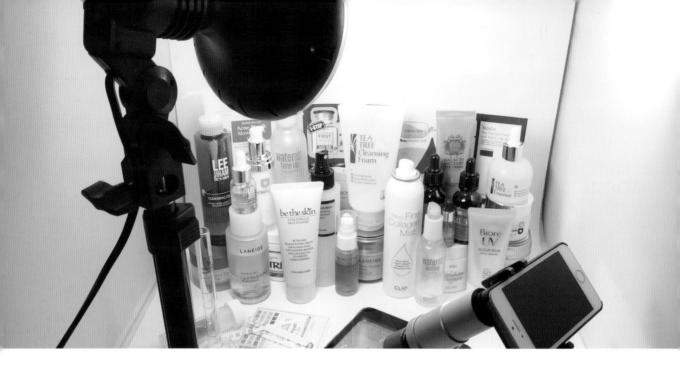

FANSERVICED-B

www.fanserviced-b.com

Fan-b details my life as an NYC-based K-beauty fangirl with oily, blemished skin. I review Korean skincare and makeup products suitable for my troubled skin, talk about products endorsed by my favorite K-pop stars, post photos from the many brick-and-mortar K-beauty stores popping up in NYC, and share shopping and Korean language resources.

SKIN TYPE
Oily and blemished, all tied firmly to hormones

SKIN CONCERNS
Hormonal acne, also acne, did I mention acne? Not destroying my skin in the process of treating said acne.

HOW I GOT INTO KOREAN BEAUTY PRODUCTS

I got into Korean beauty because the K-pop boybands I like endorse products by popular lines such as Etude House, Nature Republic, and The Saem. I went off in search of endorsement posters in NYC Korean beauty shops like Nature Republic, discovered that snail in beauty products is a thing (initially I was disgusted by this, thinking that the snails were ground up and added to the products), and accidentally fell down the rabbit hole.

MORNING SKINCARE ROUTINE

1. Foam Cleanse

I start my routine with a low-pH cleanser. I use a peanut-sized dot, add some water in order to create foam, and gently rub this onto my face. I often cradle my face in the foam and just think about how much I want to stick my head in the toilet rather than going to work.

> MY FAVORITE CLEANSER:
> *Leejiham (LJH) Tea Tree 30 Cleansing Foam*
> LJH's foaming cleanser takes the cake because it manages to get my skin clean, very-slightly moisturized, and fresh-feeling without making it squeaky and stripped.

2. pH-Adjusting Toner

The point of this step is to just take my skin from a higher pH into a range closer to exfoliation level so that acids and exfoliants can get to work on turning over cells. It's not glamorous, but it's necessary. I apply my toner with a Purederm Micro-Fiber Pad (basically a gentle, nice cotton pad) to keep from applying too much product, and to make sure that the application is even across my face. I swipe this all over and let it dry—it takes about thirty seconds to move on to the next step.

> MY CURRENT TONER:
> *COSRX AHA/BHA Clarifying Treatment Toner*
> This toner lowers my skin's pH to pave the way for the work of my vitamin C treatment. It's not terribly exciting, but the ingredient list is straightforward and simple—and it doesn't include alcohol.

3. Vitamin C/Exfoliation

Vitamin C is a recent addition to my routine. I've owned vitamin C serums for months now, but they ended up in my fridge in hopes of staving off oxidation after an initial test of both. Here's the thing about vitamin C: it will rip through your blemishes, and the necessary waiting time to let it work is a pain. I kind of love the skin destruction effect, since it means that even stubborn cystic acne is forced to have a day of reckoning and die, but there's a whole lot of drying and purging all at once. Don't start this immediately before a big event if you have acne because, seriously, your skin will be sent to Heaven whether it wants to go or not.

Vitamin C also has brightening effects and it helps with lightening hyperpigmentation left over from past blemishes. At this point I'm still riding the crazy-purge train, but my skin does look quite bright.

I apply a ton of this since I feel like my time is more valuable than the serum and I'd rather waste serum than time. I give it fifteen minutes to do its thing, spray it with some water micro mist, and then wipe off anything that wants to budge and sometimes I straight-up rinse it off in the sink.

CURRENTLY TESTING:

C20 and C21.5

C20 is an older formula that is slightly stickier and contains alcohol. C21 is newer with no alcohol and no niacinamide. Perhaps due to the alcohol, I actually find that the C20 works better for me, believe it or not. Skincare companies know that alcohol can be drying, but they sometimes choose to include it because it can increase the efficacy of the active ingredients. I'm going to continue testing both to try to determine which wins a place in my routine. It may be that my wild over-application technique will force me to go with the gentler C21.5 version.

4. Nutritious First Essence

I apply the first essence with a Purederm Micro-Fiber Pad to keep from applying too much product and to make sure that the application is even across my face. I swipe this all over and let it dry—it takes about 1 minute to move on to the next step.

Here's my feeling about oily, blemish-prone skin: once you're done with acids and prescription steps, treat it like a queen. If you're using all of that acid stuff on it, it may need some love, water, and oil to look good in the present and glow. Make the parts of your skin that don't have blemishes gorgeous right now by giving them nice things.

MY FAVORITE FIRST ESSENCE:
Goodal Waterest Tone Up First Essence
What I like about this first essence is that it not only contains fermented green tea, but also fermented oils. My skin has gotten vastly happier since I've incorporated Goodal products containing fermented oils into the start of my routine; it delivers small quantities of the rich stuff early and deeply, which is necessary since even a bit of straight oil later in my routine can make my skin grouchy and too oily looking.

5. Hydration Booster

This step is pretty specific to the Goodal line. I like the Goodal Water Oil a lot because it delivers water-based moisture and fermented oils into my skin, and also adds a moisture-grabbing gum to the surface of my skin before I apply essences.

Two pumps cover my face and dry in about two minutes, leaving my skin not exactly sticky, but sort of thirsty for the next steps. I use this to make sure that my skin is soft and fluffy even if I'm hitting it hard with a lot of exfoliants—it's super in winter, especially to prevent cold-related tightness.

THE PRODUCT I USE:
Goodal Waterest Lasting Water Oil

6. Hydrating Mist

At any point in my skincare routine when I feel like my skin is anything but dewy, I apply a hydrating micro mist. The idea is that dry skin has a harder time absorbing the things you add to your face. There's a lot of talk about applying the first post cleansing step quickly after turning from the basin in order to avoid moisture loss: using the micro-mist is a way to fake that moisturized look whenever you want.

I used to groan at mists because I thought they were fussy and annoying, but once I tried micro-mists, I saw the light. Without having to even touch your face, you can have a nutrient-rich layer of water sandwiched between your skincare layers. Sounds nice, eh? I like to apply this right after the water oil. One quick spray all over my face gets me glowing.

MY CURRENT MIST:
Clio Micro Fine Collagen Mist
This is a pretty standard micro mist with the addition of plant collagen. I'm not certain that I really need the collagen and I'd like something lighter in the future, so I'm looking to try a few other varieties to see what delivers more than just water without adding weight to my layers.

7., 8., and 9. Essences & Serums

Essences and serums are my favorite steps of all, I feel like this is where I get to slap things together like a mad chef in the kitchen. Here is where I try to target certain concerns. This is also where my skin benefits most from the genius of Korean skincare science. I like to layer just about anything related to acne treatment and healing in this step, one after the other, from lightest to heaviest in terms of thickness. This is kind of excessive, but I have a ridiculous amount of great products that my skin loves, so I go a bit wild.

THE PRODUCT I MUST USE EVERY DAY:
Leejiham (LJH) Tea Tree 90 Essence
It's been one year since I fell in love with LJH's tea tree essence and my affection for it has not waned. It's packed with good stuff for blemished skin and calms existing spots like no other. Since publishing my reviews of this essence I've heard from many people who have become addicted to this fairly light, not very moisturizing, non-astringent essence due to its magical calming properties.

10. Moisturizing Cream + Ampoules

I always try to wear a moisturizer—my hope is that by the end of my routine, my skin is balanced and happy, and still able to handle a light cream. Since I pack fermented oil and plant collagen into the early stages of my routine, I don't always need much at the end, depending on the condition of my skin and the weather. I take an almond-sized amount of cream, add one drop of ampoule, mix it together in my palm, and slather it on.

THE PRODUCTS I USE MOST OFTEN:
SN Plant Stem Cell Cream + 1 drop of Soy Bio+ Ampoule
The SN cream is miraculously good at controlling oil and providing just a bit of moisture. I mix one drop of Soy Bio+'s divine fermented soybean extract ampoule into my cream to give my skin a glow without oiliness.

11. Sunscreen

My skin gets two rounds of exfoliation, once in the morning and once at night, so it's essential that I protect all that new skin I'm exposing by applying sunscreen at the end of my morning routine. I very much prefer sunscreens that feel like proper skincare to the heavier versions made commonly outside of Asia.

THE PRODUCT I USE:
Bioré UV Aqua Rich Watery Essence SPF 50+ PA++++ (Japanese)
This sunscreen in stupidly awesome—it protects at the highest level possible, PA++++, and it actually feels good on my skin. From the moment I tried it, I was absolutely in love—it's the sunscreen for people who thought they hated sunscreen.

EVENING SKINCARE ROUTINE

1. Oil Cleanse

I start my evening routine with an oil cleanser. I've tested tons of first-step cleansers, but I really prefer oil to get all of my makeup and sunscreen off efficiently and without leaving any residue. A good first-step cleanser is important because sometimes I come home and feel like my makeup has been infiltrated by NYC's foul, sticky, black dust.

> MY FAVORITE CLEANSER:
> *Leejiham Dr's Care Cleansing Oil*
> The thing that's fantastic about this oil is that it efficiently removes makeup without leaving anything behind; other cleansing oils add moisture, but this one just banishes all the gross stuff, while adding nothing in its place. It's basically relief in a bottle.

2. Foam Cleanse

I continue with a low-pH cleanser. As far as cleansers go, I'm looking for something with a pH level that's lower than tap water. I use a peanut-sized dot, add some water in order to create foam, and gently rub this onto my face.

> MY FAVORITE CLEANSER:
> *Leejiham (LJH) Tea Tree 30 Cleansing Foam*

3. Makeup Remover

I try to get all of my makeup off by using oil, but it doesn't always play well with my contacts. I don't sweat it and just use a two-layer silicone makeup remover to wipe off all traces of my tarantula-lashes after I'm finished with my cleaning routine.

> THE PRODUCT I USE:
> *Laneige Lip and Eye Makeup Cleanser Waterproof*
> This product is so great that even I, a product junkie, happily settled down with it after trying a deluxe sample. To use it, just shake it up, apply it to a cotton pad, and swipe it away. Everything comes off without a problem—and without disturbing my contacts.

2. pH-Adjusting Toner

Same as the the pH-adjusting step from my morning routine—preparing my skin for exfoliation is equally as important in the evening.

5. BHA

My skin desperately needs BHAs—otherwise knows as salicylic acid—in order to function without having a meltdown. BHAs exfoliate the surface of skin, go in and unblock clogged pores, and are anti-inflammatory and antibacterial. After adding the right BHA to my routine, along with fermented oil skincare products, my pores begin giving up all the nasty, gritty clogs that had been hiding in there forever. Yuck. But awesome.

THE PRODUCT I USE:
Stridex Maximum Strength (North American)
I never considered using Stridex until hearing about it from other skincare fans—it always seemed way too "high school jock boy drying his face with alcohol" to me. It turns out it is exactly what my face needed: a straight shot of serious 2% salicylic acid (with no alcohol) that isn't excessively drying to my skin and adds no residue.

6. Prescription Medication

Prescription medication is something I added to my routine about nine months ago, and it's been good, but it's still not enough to overcome the war of hormones going on inside. I use it consistently, to clear my pores of old grime and create a net that catches anything that's caused by my envioronment. I apply two to three pumps of this, carefully avoiding my eyes and mouth and then make sure it gets a solid forty-five minutes to do its thing in peace.

THE PRESCRIPTION I USE:
Pocketderm: 0.04% Tretinoin, 1% Clindamycin, 7% Azelaic Acid
Tretinoin is like a skin-cell life coach, clindamycin is an antibiotic, and azelaic acid helps to heal acne caused by bacteria. I like the Pocketderm service because I'm lazy and this just gets mailed to me; if prescription acne medication were any more difficult to get, I'd probably just skip it.

7. Either Fall Asleep or Continue with Essence

Forty-five minutes is a long time to wait at night for my prescription medication to work. Since Pocketderm's formula contains moisturizers, I'm a-okay with collapsing into my pillow and going to sleep after I apply it. If I'm feeling more awake, or if I started my routine earlier, I'll continue with the one essential essence in my stash. My skin likes it a whole lot more if I stay up late to pamper it, but ultimately the needs of my brain come before the needs of my brain's container.

MY FAVORITE ESSENCE:
Leejiham (LJH) Tea Tree 90 Essence

8. Cream or Sleeping Pack with Optional Ampoule

Nighttime is fun because it's when I can bust out some lovely products that would result in oil-related disasters if I use them during the day. Sometimes I pick a cream and at other times a sleeping pack. What's the difference? Uhhh...the name?

THE CREAMS & PACKS I USE:
Migabee Beevenom and Honey Cream
The Migabee cream is great even during the day, but it lacks the oil-controlling properties of my favorite for-daytime wear, so it's a special treat at bedtime.

Laneige Water Sleeping Pack
The Laneige Sleeping Pack is a bit sticky on my face at bedtime, but I wake up with the most incredibly soft, smooth skin.

THE AMPOULES I USE:
Su:m 37 Losec Therapy
Leejiham (LJH) Propolis Ampoule
I like to use rich ampoules at bedtime. One drop turns my face into a glorious, goopy mess, but helps my skin heal faster and look better in the morning.

9. Eye Cream

I can't believe that I use an eye cream. Urgh, what have I become?! That's not very punk rock! I should just be able to use one of the ten million stupid creams I own, but of course, I need an eye cream. A good, non-comedogenic eye cream means the difference of five to ten years in terms of my appearance. I have what's called an "eye smile" in Korea, or what researchers call a *Duchenne smile*, meaning that my eyes squint when I smile. And I smile a *lot* because I walk around most of the day cracking (mostly inappropriate) jokes, even if I'm the only one in the room. The only downside to an eye smile is that it means my face is constantly creasing from all that smiling. My goal is to have people who have been corresponding with me by email look at my face when we meet and assume that I couldn't possibly be the person they've been talking to, because I look like I'm only old enough to be my own assistant. Most of the time, it works. Thank you, eye cream, for making things awkward at work a few times per year.

THE PRODUCT I USE:
Purebess Galactomyces Eye Cream 80
This stuff is what changed my mind about eye cream—it's dirt cheap, poses no problems for my skin, and it gently hydrates my delicate eye skin without making it greasy. It's my pick for the K-beauty product that could make anyone a believer.

10. Blemish Patches

I consider blemish patches to be essential tools for any blemish-sufferer. Despite our best attempts, sometimes bad things happen. By bad things I, of course, mean blemishes. Blemish patches, depending on their quality level, can protect your skin from your picky fingers, keep blemishes open so that they can gently drain their inner garbage, encourage blemishes to come to a head, and encourage whitehead blemishes to open without causing them trauma. They're really great wound care and something I think should be given out in high school health classes because they're so game-changing.

HIGH-END BLEMISH PATCHES I USE:
COSRX Acne Pimple Master Patch
The COSRX patches are the right balance between sticky and removable, and they are

true hydrocolloid bandage patches. Upon waking up, if I've put the COSRX patches on the right blemishes, there will be moisture trapped right in the patch and a flattened blemish head left behind.

BUDGET-FRIENDLY BLEMISH PATCHES I USE:
A'Pieu Nonco Tea Tree Spot Patch
The A'Pieu patches are less dramatic, but they're about one-tenth the cost, but I think they do more than one-tenth the work, and are therefore worth mentioning! They are rather thin discs that do most of the functions of the COSRX patches —except extract liquid from blemishes.

SPECIAL CARE

Sheet Masks
I am very much *not* in the one-a-day sheet mask club. I find that most of the ingredients in my other products are superior to those in the sheet masks, so I save them for occasions when I need a hydration jolt.

MY FAVORITES:
Enesti Aloe Multi Care Mask
The Enesti is a basic-as-hell sheet mask that's just really good at delivering moisture while being super comfortable to wear; I often use these when traveling because the mask fabric is thick and cozy, somehow lulling me to sleep easily.

Mediental Snail Aquaring SOS Mask
The Mediental mask is a two-step mask: the creamy pre treatment essence is applied first, followed by application of an essence-soaked sheet mask. What makes this mask exceptional is the zero-irritation or pain that results from this mask.

Physical Exfoliation

Given my regular and serious chemical exfoliation on a daily basis, I am very careful about not over-exfoliating my skin using physical means like brushes and scrubs. About once per week, I use a peeling gel/treatment that doesn't really peel my face, but rather clears skin build-up, and takes away dead skin flakes.

THE PRODUCT I USE:

Be the Skin Non-Stimulus Face Polisher

I'm a big fan of gommage or peeling gels, and this one takes the cake—it exfoliates fantastically, removes excess oil, smells pretty good. It's so addictive that I have to stop myself from using it too often, for fear that I'll overexfoliate and thin-out my skin.

Repairing Treatment

Sometimes, whether it's due to overdrying from acids and prescriptions or, say, a runny nose, our faces get chapped and dry far beyond the normal bounds. Thankfully, there's a cream for that.

THE PRODUCT I USE:

Laneige Multiberry Yogurt Pack

This repair pack is meant to be a twenty-five-minute wash-off mask treatment, but I've certainly used it as an overnight mask on truly distressed skin. It heals even chapped-to-the-point-of-bleeding skin and it doesn't cause me to break out. It's like a lovely, less repulsive version of Vaseline.

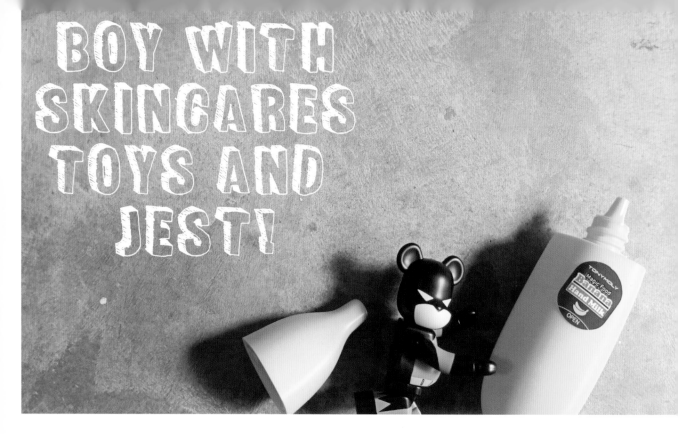

RYANRAROAR

www.ryanraroar.com

I share with readers everything about beauty and my personal take on it. My blog shows you what's new, what's exciting, as well as products I have tried, loved, and reviewed from an Asian perspective.

SKIN TYPE

Combination skin type that is acne-prone and speckled with post-acne-marks and scars. My T-zone is oilier and have issues with blackheads and shine.

SKIN CONCERNS

Recurring pimples, clogged pores, shiny T-zone, post-acne marks and scars, and dark circles.

THE K-BEAUTY PHILOSOPHY THAT RESONATES WITH ME

The inspiration for many Korean beauty products stems from ancient literature that has been passed down through the generations. This literature identifies various ingredients and their skincare benefits. I buy into the wisdom and ideals that have worked so beautifully since the Joseon period. This wisdom, coupled with the latest technology and innovations, has proved to be a winning combo.

I also like that each product can perform beautifully on its own, or in harmony with an entire skincare line. This encourages users to be creative and customize a routine using only the products that work best for them. After all, every skin type is unique.

MORNING SKINCARE ROUTINE

1. Cleanse

Choosing the right type of cleanser is important, as it will ensure minimal irritation and disruption to your skin's natural balance.

MY PREFERRED CLEANSERS:
COSRX Salicylic Acid Exfoliating Cleanser
TonyMoly Aquaporin Moisture Foam Cleanser

2. Tone

I especially love using the COSRX AHA/BHA Clarifying Treatment Toner because of its daily mild exfoliating action. It aids in cell renewal and promotes clearer skin.

MY FAVORITE TONER:
COSRX AHA / BHA Clarifying Treatment Toner

3. Treat (Ampoule + Serum/Essence)

Ampoules are especially important as they contain a higher percentage of active ingredients that deliver the needed effect. I really like CNP Laboratory Mugener Ampule, which calms skin redness and spots.

Serums and essence are like your daily maintenance tools for keeping your skin in tip-top condition. When my skin looks dull and lifeless, the Naruko Rose & Botanic HA Aqua Cubic Complex EX always seems to whip it back into shape.

MY PREFERRED AMPOULE:
CNP Laboratory Mugener Ampule

MY PREFERRED SERUM/ESSENCE:
Naruko Rose & Botanic HA Aqua Cubic Complex EX

4. Eye Care

If you keep your eye area moist and healthy, your eyes will always sparkle! This is because wrinkles and fine lines look less harsh when the skin surface is moist. For that reason, I love using the TonyMoly Floria Whitening Eye Serum; it comes with a metal-tip applicator that provides an immediate, cooling, and soothing effect.

MY FAVORITE EYE TREATMENT:
TonyMoly Floria Whitening Eye Serum

5. Moisturize

Since I have a combination/acne-prone skin type, I always go for moisturizers with a light and fast-absorbing texture. The snail cream from TonyMoly is especially refreshing, its gel-creme form absorbs quickly and provides a plethora of benefits such as healing, redness reduction, and hydration. On days my skin is feeling dry or flaky, I will mix in a few drops of facial oil to amp up the moisture.

MY FAVORITE MOISTURIZER:
TonyMoly Intense Care Gold 24K Snail Cream

6. Sun Protection

The single most important product everyone needs is sunscreen. For my combination/acne-prone skin type, I go for something light and refreshing.

MY PREFERRED SUNSCREENS:
Dr.Wu UV Protective Cream with Tinosorb M (Tinted) SPF50 PA+++
Bioré UV Aqua Rich Watery Essence SPF50+ PA++++ (Japanese)

7. Base Makeup

When I have a breakout, I count on the calming and oil-controlling benefits of TonyMoly Tony Lab AC Control BB Cream to bring in additional acne-fighting help, it also conceals imperfections.

MY BASE MAKEUP PICK:
TonyMoly Tony Lab AC Control BB Cream SPF30 PA++

8. Mist

I carry a small bottle of facial mist with me so that I can freshen up my skin any time of the day. Face mist offers an immediate cooling and hydrating effect, and the fact that it works well over the makeup is awesome.

MY FACIAL MIST PICKS:
Innisfree Green Tea Mineral Mist
CremorLab T.E.N Cremor Mineral Water

EVENING SKINCARE ROUTINE

1. Pre-cleanse (Remove Makeup)

Because I wear lighter makeup, I simply use a cleansing wipe for this step. I especially like the Bifesta Cleansing Express Bright Up Cleansing Sheet because each piece is soaked with sufficient cleansing liquid that effortlessly removes all traces of makeup. No scrubbing at all!

Bifesta Cleansing Express Bright Up Cleansing Sheet (Japanese)

2. Cleanse

As is the case with my morning cleanse, it is important that my evening cleanse will prevent irritation and/or disruption to my skin's natural balance.

MY PREFERRED CLEANSERS:
COSRX Salicylic Acid Exfoliating Cleanser
TonyMoly Aquaporin Moisture Foam Cleanser

3. Exfoliate

Exfoliate regularly to remove dead skin cells, and to prevent blackheads and pimples from forming. Do not scrub if you have pimples that are inflamed, as it will irritate the skin! Generally, I exfoliate twice a week. However, if I have a chemical peel or microdermabrasion done, I will skip the home exfoliation. I use the Kiehl's Epidermal Re-Texturizing Micro-Dermabrasion to give my skin a deep exfoliation and prep it for the next-step skincare.

MY PREFERRED EXFOLIATOR:
Kiehl's Epidermal Re-Texturizing Micro-Dermabrasion (U.S. American)

4. Tone

I especially love using the COSRX AHA/BHA Clarifying Treatment Toner because of its daily, mild-exfoliating action. It aids in cell renewal and promotes clearer skin.

MY FAVORITE TONER:
COSRX AHA / BHA Clarifying Treatment Toner

5. Mask

If your skin is normal and you want to do a hydrating mask every day, go for it. But if your skin is oily or acne-prone, stick to doing a mask two or three times a week to prevent overburdening your reactive skin. Always stick to the recommended duration and never overdo it. I simply love doing the Mamonde Lotus Micro Mud Mask because, unlike most mud or clay masks, it does not over-dry skin, and it offers sebum-regulating and pore-purifying benefits at the same time.

MY PREFERRED MASK:
Mamonde Lotus Micro Mud Mask

6. Treat (Ampoule + Serum/Essence)

I use the same ampoule and serum in my evening routine to keep my skin in its ideal state.

MY PREFERRED AMPOULE:
CNP Laboratory Mugener Ampule

MY PREFERRED SERUM/ESSENCE:
Naruko Rose & Botanic HA Aqua Cubic Complex EX

7. Eye Care

I never skip eye care in the evening—keeping my eye area nourished while I sleep is essential if I want to wake up to youthful, sparkling eyes.

MY FAVORITE EYE TREATMENT:
TonyMoly Floria Whitening Eye Serum

8. Moisturize

My evening moisturizer choice is the same as the one I use in my morning routine. It provides the same refreshing hydrating benefits at night as it does during the day.

MY FAVORITE MOISTURIZER:
TonyMoly Intense Care Gold 24K Snail Cream

9. Targeted Treatment

Choose a spot treatment that does not dry skin, or risk making the spot even angrier. I rely on Clinique Acne Solution Spot Healing Gel to clear up the inflammation and prevent scarring.

10. Sleeping Mask

A sleeping mask offers an entire night of treatment and moisture that is important even for acne sufferers. The trick is to choose one that is light and refreshing, and not the heavier, nourishing type, which is better for drier or mature skin. Because of its ability to heal and comfort pimples, I enjoy using the Missha Super Aqua Cell Renew Snail Sleeping Mask once a week.

MY FAVORITE SLEEPING MASK:
Missha Super Aqua Cell Renew Snail Sleeping Mask

11. Lip Care

The skin on the lips is significantly thinner than the skin on the rest of your face. Nourishing the lips is important, especially if you wear lots of lip makeup. The makeup removal process can have a detrimental effect on the lips, and the constant wiping and tugging the cotton balls can cause unwanted wrinkles. To combat this, use a nourishing lip-care product every night to condition the lips. I swear by the Rosebud Perfume Co. Menthol and Eucalyptus Balm. It has a thick texture to coat my lips in a protective film, which prevents moisture from evaporating as I sleep the night away in an air-conditioned room.

MY PREFERRED LIP TREATMENT:
Rosebud Perfume Co. Menthol and Eucalyptus Balm (U.S. American)

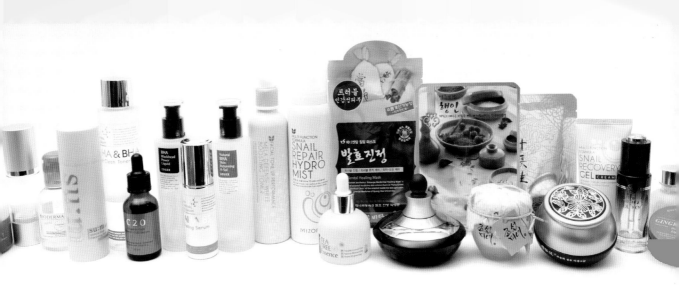

SNOW WHITE & THE ASIAN PEAR

snowwhiteandthepear.blogspot.com

I'm a melanin-challenged Canadian girl who learned to embrace her natural skin tone through discovering the world of Asian beauty products. I have typical can't-tan-just-burn skin, and I live in the desert, so it can be a challenge to keep skin healthy and glowing instead of looking like sun-scorched, desiccated leather. At the time I started my blog, Asian product reviews were hard to find, and now here we are: full of Hanbang, science, and snails.

SKIN TYPE
Dehydrated, combination skin—oily with dry cheeks

SKIN CONCERNS
Congested pores, acne-prone, hyperpigmentation, sun damage, aging

CLIMATE

Arid with high winds, high temperatures, and large amounts of dust/dirt in the air. Frequent *haboobs* (dust/sandstorms) and herds of migrating tumbleweeds.

HOW I FOUND THE WAY OF THE SNAIL

More than anything else, it was moving from Canada to a desert that catalyzed my Korean skincare journey. Predictably, it was a disaster. It was another planet! How did I wind up on the set of Arrakis?! Lightning inside of dust storms. Cacti and mesquite. Summer for more than ten months out of the year. The sun sears the earth, and anyone on it, with a palpable force of heat akin to standing next to a wood stove on a cold night, but with an eye-scalding brightness that makes your retinas beg for mercy even in the cold depths of January. In five years, my face looked *twenty* years older, but my skin hated sunscreen with the burning passion of a thousand pores. That's when I discovered BB creams, and then Korean skincare (and snails), which solved my skin issues. At the time, my skin was oily, yet dry all at once, pebbled by clogged pores and littered with dry flakes. Customization is a wonderful, wonderful thing.

The Korean skincare approach has allowed me the flexibility to address my skin's diverse needs and petulant moods. I can have it all: anti-acne alongside anti-aging, hydration without heaviness, and a routine as simple, or complex, as I need at that moment.

MY SKINCARE ROUTINE

My routine is an ever-shifting, ever-rotating, expanding-and-contracting lineup of Western and Asian skincare, with an overwhelmingly Korean-product population. The beauty of the multi-step and customized approach is about finding the right product for the task, no matter what the product's origins are, but I can't deny that Korea has it all down to an art.

I have some core products that are staples in my routine, but my routine is primarily based around step/function, rather than specific products. I add in or swap various products depending on how my skin feels, and many of the products featured in the photos are simply what I am using now, and will be replaced with others as I use them up.

My routine, no matter how flexible and transient it may be, can be boiled down to these basic steps, in this order:

1. Cleansers
2. Actives
3. Hydrators
4. Occlusives
5. Treatments/Sun Protection

I might use only a single product from each step, or many, depending on my skin's condition at the moment. Listening to your skin is the best advice I can give to someone contemplating how to build their routine; identify your skin's needs and then select products that fit those needs.

1. Cleansers

As someone with clog-prone skin in a dusty environment, I need to thoroughly cleanse and rinse my skin to keep breakouts at bay. I double-cleanse with an oil-type makeup-removing cleanser, followed by a low-pH foaming cleanser to remove residue.

MAKEUP REMOVING CLEANSER:
(PM) *Leejiham Dr's Care Cleansing Oil*
Used as a first cleanser and also as a massage oil to clear my pores.

CLEANSING WATER:
(AM) *Bioderma Crealine H2O Solution Micellaire (French)*
Although cleansing waters haven't proved effective as a makeup removing-cleanser for me, I love them for a gentle AM cleanse when my skin doesn't need a full-foaming cleanser.

FACIAL CLEANSER:
(AM/PM) *Su:m37 Miracle Rose Cleansing Stick*
Used daily as a primary cleanser, or as a second cleanser after removing makeup and sunscreen. Low-pH, gentle, and suffused with rose oil and petals.

2. Actives

Actives are where skincare magic happens in earnest. I use a pH-adjusting toner to prep my skin, and then a lineup of heavy-hitters which can include vitamin C serums, BHA exfoliants, AHA exfoliants, and acne treatments. I use vitamin C for anti-aging and fading pigmentation, BHA for clearing my pores, and AHA for fading pigmentation, improving skin texture, and keeping those pesky dry patches away.

> PH-ADJUSTING TONER:
> *(AM/PM) Mizon AHA/BHA Daily Clean Toner*
> A staple for me and the most gentle pH-adjusting toner I have used. It lets me skip the wait-time between cleansing and actives, preventing my skin from drying out between those steps.

> VITAMIN C SERUM:
> *(AM) OST C20 Original Pure Vitamin C20 Serum*

> BHA EXFOLIANT:
> *(AM/PM) COSRX BHA Blackhead Power Liquid*
> This treatment is so gentle that I can use it daily if I feel like my skin needs it.

> AHA EXFOLIANT:
> *(PM) Mizon 8% AHA Peeling Serum*
> Used one to three times a week, as needed.

> ACNE TREATMENT:
> *(AM/PM) COSRX Natural BHA Skin Returning A-Sol*
> Used as an acne treatment, this product contains a small amount of BHA and AHA, and a large amount of propolis.

3. Hydrators

As a desert dweller, replenishing the water in my skin is a top priority. Ensuring I have hydrated my skin before adding products containing oil keeps my skin balanced throughout the day. I use a bevy of mists, hydrating toners, essences, serums, ampoules, and sheet masks (even at times in the AM) to restore my skin's balance.

HYDRATING TONER:
(AM/PM) Mizon Mela Defense White Boosting Toner
Used only if I want to wipe off leftover residue from my actives step, including exfoliated dead skin. If I can feel balled-up, dead skin under my fingers, I like to wipe that off before I apply other products.

MIST:
(AM/PM) Mizon Snail Repair Hydro Mist
Used if my skin feels a bit dry after actives, to cool my face, or throughout the day to boost hydration without disrupting my sunscreen or makeup. I even mist the puff from my makeup cushions before picking up product for extra hydration during application.

ESSENCE/SERUM:
(AM/PM) Leejiham Tea Tree 90 Essence
Uses the tea tree extract, which is much gentler than the oil; this lovely anti-acne serum is a staple of my lineup that I use it twice a day.

(AM/PM) Sooryehan Hyo Biyeon Concentrated Brightening Essence
Currently the "product undergoing testing" in my lineup. Begone, hyperpigmentation!

SHEET MASK:
(AM/PM) Varies, used daily or sometimes twice a day. I am particularly fond of *hanbang* (traditional Korean herbal medicine) products and sheet masks are no exception; the Mediental and Evercos masks are two of my favorites! Daily sheet masks are not for everyone, but I need all the sustained moisture I can get.

4. Occlusives

As someone with dehydrated skin, as opposed to dry skin, I apply occlusive products very sparingly. Occlusives act as a barrier, sealing hydration into the skin, and are often rich, oily, or heavy in silicones. I also use them only in the areas I need, because overloading my skin with rich products leads to clogged pores and breakouts.

LIGHT CREAM:
(AM/PM) *Mizon Multi Function Formula Snail Recovery Gel Cream*
Used if it's a hot day, during the summer, or any time I feel I need something ultra light on my skin instead of a traditional cream. This product was my first ever Korean skincare purchase, and four years and many tubes later, it is still a staple.

MEDIUM CREAM:
(AM/PM) *Beauty of Joseon Dynasty Cream*
Used in all seasons when I want something robust enough to keep my skin supple and moisturized for hours. It's also my current favorite product.

HEAVY CREAM:
(AM/PM) *Buyonghwa Princess Jeonghyo Wild Cream*
Used only in winter, or when my skin is feeling very dry.

FACIAL OIL:
(PM) *Hankook Cosmetics The Prestige Gold Oil Essence*
Used only when I feel I need to boost my cream with the added richness of an oil.

4. Sun Protection (AM)

I work indoors in front of two large windows. Therefore, sunscreen is a must whether I am inside or outside, but my skin will not tolerate chemical UV filters. I rely on physical sunscreens, and I am still searching for that One True Love. I wear a lower-rated sunscreen indoors, and boost up the protection if I go outside. Working from home has its perks; if I need to give my skin a break from sunscreen, I can close the blinds and work from the sunless comfort of my bat cave.

INDOOR SUNSCREEN:

IOPE UV Shield Sun Mild Clinic SPF25 PA++

Used on days I do not need a strong protection from outdoor exposure.

OUTDOOR SUNSCREEN:

Sunkiller Baby Milk SPF45 PA+++

Used on days I go outside during the day; cannot be worn under makeup and has a strong white cast.

5. Treatments (PM)

SPOT TREATMENT:

Mizon Acence Blemish Out Pink Spot

Used on developing blemishes that I want to hasten along in deciding whether they are going to disappear or come to a head.

3M Nexcare Blemish Clear Cover Hydrocolloid Bandages

A staple in my lineup. When applied to an open blemish, they safely, gently, and hygienically drain it, leaving it flattened and partially healed in a fraction of the normal time.

LIP TREATMENT:

Aritaum Ginger Sugar Overnight Lip Mask

Used when my lips feel dry. I developed the habit of licking my lips before sneezing because they would split when I did, which was quite painful! Now my lips are supple and soft when I wake up.

CLAY MASK:

Innisfree Jeju Volcanic Pore Clay Mask

Used one to two times a month. Clay masks can be quite drying, so I use this primarily to kickstart loosening clogged pores before an oil massage.

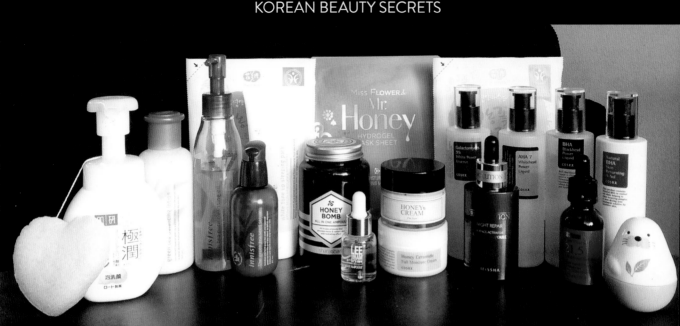

FIFTY SHADES OF SNAIL

www.fiftyshadesofsnail.com

Blogger and Fashionista.com K-beauty correspondent, Jude Chao writes a beauty blog dedicated to helping readers of all ages, skin types, and budgets achieve beautiful skin through Asian skincare rituals and routines. With extensive product reviews, industry features, ingredient analyses, and skincare tips, tricks, and tutorials, *Fifty Shades of Snail* aims to help both skincare newbies and hardcore addicts discover the best products for their needs.

SKIN TYPE
Normal/balanced, nonreactive

SKIN CONCERNS
Brightening, firming, minimizing effects of photoaging. The vast majority of my routine aims to repair past sun damage and prevent future sun damage.

WHY I LOVE K-BEAUTY

My love for K-beauty is more than skin deep. I never achieved truly great results with Western products, nor was I ever particularly attracted to them. The Korean aesthetic and the beauty standards that Korean brands target are much more closely aligned with my personal tastes, and I find the ritualistic nature of the Korean skincare regimen meditative and soothing. In fact, although Korean skincare products have improved my skin by leaps and bounds in the two years since I started on this journey, the Korean skincare routine has improved my mental health even more.

MORNING SKINCARE ROUTINE

1. Foaming Cleanser:
Hada Labo Gokujyun Hyaluronic Acid Cleansing Foam (Japanese)
I like to gently but thoroughly cleanse my skin in the morning and sweep away any dead skin loosened during the night to prepare it for my morning treatment steps and to create the best canvas for makeup.

2. Toner:
COSRX Natural BHA Skin Returning A-Sol, mixed with one drop of *LeeJiham (LJH) Vita Propolis Ampoule*
The propolis extract contained in both these products, as well as the botanical extracts in the LJH ampoule, deliver a high dose of healing and protective antioxidants to prepare for the day's UV and pollution exposure.

3. Essence:
COSRX Galactomyces 95 White Power Essence
Combines galactomyces ferment extract with niacinamide and humectants to brighten, firm, and hydrate skin.

4. Ampoules:

Shara Shara Honey Bomb All In One Ampoule
Blends the moisturizing, reparative, and protective properties of honey and propolis with more brightening niacinamide and hydrating humectants to further soften and plump skin.

Missha Time Revolution Night Repair Science Activator Borabit Ampoule
Repairs past sun damage and helps protect against future free-radical damage with a potent mix of antioxidants, proven anti-aging actives, and plant and ferment extracts.

5. Serum:

Innisfree Green Tea Seed Serum
Further protects skin with a combination of green tea and other botanical antioxidants, and delivers one last dose of humectant hydration to help make sure skin stays moist all day long.

6. Emulsion:

Innisfree Green Tea Balancing Lotion
Lightly seals in the morning's treatment steps with a fast-absorbing, non-oily texture that plays well with sunscreen and makeup.

7. Sunscreen:

Bioré UV Aqua Rich Watery Essence SPF 50+ PA++++ (Japanese)
Protects skin against UV damage with high UVB and UVA protection and a light, natural, matte finish.

EVENING SKINCARE ROUTINE

1. Oil Cleanser:

Innisfree Green Tea Pure Cleansing Oil
Quickly breaks up and lifts off the day's makeup, sunscreen, oil, dirt, and sweat.

2. Foaming Cleanser:

Hada Labo Gokujyun Hyaluronic Acid Cleansing Foam (Japanese)

3. Vitamin C Serum:

C21.5 Pure Vitamin C Serum, mixed with a drop of *LeeJiham (LJH) Vita Propolis Ampoule*
Gives skin a potent dose of propolis, niacinamide, antioxidants, and L-ascorbic acid to lighten old sunspots, repair UV damage, and boost barrier function and collagen production.

4. BHA:

COSRX BHA Blackhead Power Liquid
Gently but thoroughly clears sebum and dead skin cells out from pores, helping them stay clean and unclogged.

5. AHA:

COSRX AHA 7 Whitehead Power Liquid
Gently and gradually exfoliates dead cells from the surface of skin, smoothing, and brightening its appearance and minimizing fine lines and wrinkles.

6. Toner:

COSRX Natural BHA Skin Returning A-Sol

7. Essence:

COSRX Galactomyces 95 White Power Essence

8. Ampoule:

Shara Shara Honey Bomb All In One Ampoule
Missha Time Revolution Night Repair Science Activator Borabit Ampoule

9. Serum:

Innisfree Green Tea Seed Serum

10. Mask:

Any one of a variety of sheet masks and hydrogel masks to deliver intensive hydration, as well as botanical extracts and/or proven actives for the rapid treatment of skin issues.

11. Cream:

I'm From Honey Cream
When skin feels dry.

COSRX Honey Ceramide Full Moisture Cream
When skin feels normal.

Both creams offer deep nourishment and emollient moisture to help skin stay moist and repair itself through the night.

12. Sleeping Pack:

Innisfree White Tone Up Sleeping Pack
A light-textured occlusive gel, infused with antioxidant botanical extracts, vitamin C, and niacinamide to brighten the complexion and seal in moisture and treatment actives overnight.

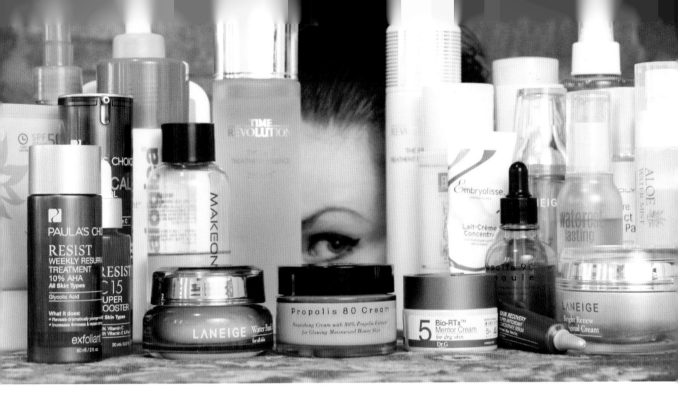

HELLO PRETTY BIRD!

www.helloprettybird.com

Hello Pretty Bird! is a beauty and lifestyle blog with a budget-conscious focus. The site features a mixture of product reviews, tutorials, and posts about other things that make life easier or more fun (like food, affordable accessories, and cheap things to do in New York City). On the beauty side of things, you'll see lots of drugstore, niche, and Asian cosmetics reviews on the site—the goal is to help folks discover new brands to love, figure out which mainstream budget products actually work, and which mid-priced (and up) products are worth the splurge.

SKIN TYPE:
Combination skin. More dry/dehydrated in the winter, oily in the T-zone in the summer.

SKIN CONCERNS:
Acne prevention, dehydration, reducing the appearance of fine lines and wrinkles.

THOUGHTS ON THE KOREAN SKINCARE PHILOSOPHY

I struggled with a typical American-style skincare routine for a long time: wash your face once, slap on some astringent toner to dry out your acne (which totally doesn't work, by the way), apply a single moisturizing cream that might be too light for some situations and too rich for others, and wonder why your skin feels like crap.

I really appreciate the layered, moisture-happy approach to skincare that Korean-style routines offer because it's easy to customize and add or remove products as demanded by the needs of your skin. Even better, there are tons of effective Korean products that are also very affordable. I'm a total cheapskate, so I appreciate that level of accessibility.

MORNING SKINCARE ROUTINE

1. Foaming Cleanser

The first step of my skincare day is to wash off my night creams, sweat and other face gunk with a gentle foaming cleanser.

> MY PERSONAL FAVORITE:
> *CeraVe Foaming Facial Cleanser (U.S. American)*
> It cleanses well without leaving skin feeling stripped, plus it's bargain-priced. I'd rather scrimp a little on cleansers so I can spend more on leave-on treatments!

2. First Treatment Essence

Once my face is nice and clean, I immediately apply a bit of treatment essence with my hands.

> MY PREFERRED FIRST TREATMENT ESSENCE:
> *Missha Time Revolution The First Treatment Essence Intensive*
> This is a lightweight, yeasty essence with slightly hydrating properties. It's a staple in my routine mainly because it softens my skin and reduces redness. I use a retinol serum as part of my nighttime routine, and this stuff calms my skin down afterwards.

3. Toner

Next I'll apply a light layer of toner. Just to clarify, I mean hydrating toner, not astringent toner. The toner category can be a bit confusing because they tend to go by many names, and they vary a lot in terms of viscosity.

> MY PERSONAL FAVORITE:
> *Rohto Hada Labo Gokujyn Hyaluronic Acid Lotion (Japanese)*
> This is a thick, slippery toner that's loaded up with hyaluronic acid. A little bit goes a long way with this stuff, but it's a huge help in keeping my skin looking supple and moisturized.

4. Serum/Ampoule

After applying toner, I immediately follow up with a few drops of an active-rich, hydrating serum or ampoule for extra glow.

> MY FAVORITES:
> *Laneige Water Bank Moisture Serum*
> *Goodal Waterest Lasting Water Oil*
> *LeeJiHam (LJH) Vita Propolis Ampoule*

All of them give skin a supple-looking radiance without making your face feel too heavy or look too oily.

5. Emulsion/Milk

Next, I follow up with a little bit of emulsion for one last moisturizing kick and to lock all the previous layers in.

> MY FAVORITE:
> *Rohto Hada Labo Gokujyun Moisture Milk (Japanese)*
> This is a total staple for me in this department because it's light and non-greasy enough to not make my makeup slide around. Nobody wants slidy makeup!

6. Sunscreen

You know what's really good for your skin? Avoiding sun damage! I'm also really, really pale and prone to sunburn, so a good sunscreen is a must. These days, I mostly prefer mineral sunscreens over chemical ones because they seem to irritate my skin less, and them being non-greasy is essential. Remember, slidy makeup = bad.

MY PICKS:
Paula's Choice Resist Super-Light Wrinkle Defense SPF 30 (U.S. American)
My everyday "I'm going to be outside walking to the subway for 10 minutes" type SPF product. It feels super-light, as the name might suggest.

Innisfree Eco Safety Perfect Waterproof Sunblock SPF50+ PA+++
For days when I'll be spending a lot of time in the sun, I try to choose something a bit stronger—this one is great because it doesn't wear off easily.

EVENING SKINCARE ROUTINE

1. Point Makeup Remover

True story: I wear a lot of waterproof eye makeup and bright lipstick. While many facial cleansers are capable of getting off stubborn makeup on their own, they're not really as efficient (or non-irritating) as using a bit of makeup remover on a soft cotton pad. I'm a big fan of dual-phase removers (the kind with two layers that you have to shake up).

MY PICKS:
Makeon Nothing Is Impossible Remover Liquid
My favorite makeup remover because of how quickly it dissolves waterproof makeup.

Neutrogena Oil Free Eye Makeup Remover (U.S. American)
A great, budget-friendly alternative that can be found in most drugstores.

2. Oil Cleanser

Discovering oil cleansers was one of the biggest game-changers for me in terms of skincare. Have you ever washed your face, rubbed it on a towel, only to leave behind makeup streaks? Ewww. That was me, every day. Now I massage a bit of oil cleanser onto my dry face and it dissolves all of my foundation/sunscreen residue like magic.

MY FAVORITE:
Innisfree Apple Juicy Cleansing Oil
It smells delicious and removes makeup thoroughly without leaving behind greasy residue.

3. Foaming Cleanser

At this point, my face is mostly clean, but I like to do one final swoop with foaming cleanser to get off any last bits of oil and makeup residue. Enter CeraVe Foaming Facial Cleanser again.

MY PERSONAL FAVORITE:
CeraVe Foaming Facial Cleanser (U.S. American)

4. Exfoliation

Exfoliation has also been a game-changer for me in terms of reducing acne and improving the texture of my skin, particularly since I started using chemical exfoliants. It's also the most complicated stage of my skincare routine because I rotate several products throughout the week to avoid overdoing it. A typical week might look something like this:

MONDAY/WEDNESDAY/FRIDAY:
Paula's Choice Skin Perfecting 2% BHA Liquid Exfoliant
This is a salicylic acid treatment that has been really helpful for me in terms of reducing acne.

TUESDAY/THURSDAY/SATURDAY:
Paula's Choice Clinical 1% Retinol Treatment
OST C20 Vitamin C Serum

I usually apply the vitamin C serum first, wait twenty minutes, then apply the retinol. The retinol seems to have a skin-smoothing effect with consistent usage (bye bye, fine lines!) and the vitamin C has been really useful for reducing post-acne marks and generally brightening my skin.

SUNDAY:
Paula's Choice Resist Weekly Resurfacing Treatment w/ 10% AHA (U.S. American)
This is probably my favorite of all the chemical treatments I use, but it's too strong to use more than once or twice per week. It's an anti-aging treatment which makes my skin look super-smooth and glowy the next day.

OCCASIONALLY:
SkinFood Black Sugar Wash-Off Mask
Kuan Yuan Lian Mung Bean Powder
Once in a while, I will skip my usual slew of chemicals and opt for a scrub instead. There isn't really any strong advantage to doing this from what I can tell, but it feels nice! The trick is to choose a scrub that's really gentle.

4. Toner

If I'm using a chemical exfoliant, I wait about fifteen to twenty minutes for acids to neutralize before doing this step.

MY PERSONAL FAVORITE:
Rohto Hada Labo Gokujyn Hyaluronic Acid Lotion (Japanese)

5. Serum/Ampoule

I'm more likely to apply these liberally at night because I don't have to worry about slidy makeup. I also find myself less concerned about a sticky ampoule if I just use it at night.

I LIKE:
Pure Heals Propolis Ampoule
Works well for hydration and giving skin that special glow.

5. Emulsion/Milk

Just like during the day, I apply a emulsion after my ampoule. I sometimes skip this step during warmer weather, because my face gets a lot oilier in the summer and that extra layer can be a bit much to handle.

MY FAVORITE:
Rohto Hada Labo Gokujyun Moisture Milk (Japanese)

8. Eye Cream

I don't like super rich creams in my eye area, because some give me milia seeds. Gel-type creams are the answer!

MY PICKS:
Laneige's Water Bank Eye Gel
Dr. Jart+ V7 Eye Serum

9. Cream

At long last, the crown atop my skincare head: cream! I use some pretty strong exfoliants at night, so I need something a bit thicker and more occlusive than emulsion to keep my skin from freaking out.

My skin gets really dry and flaky in the winter due to our savage indoor heating system, so I tend to reach for richer creams around that time of year. In the summer, I use creams that are a bit more gel-like in consistency so my skin doesn't feel totally smothered.

MY WINTER PICKS:
Laneige Water Bank Moisture Cream
Dr.G Bio-RTxTM Mentor Cream #5

MY SUMMER PICKS:
Pure Heals Propolis Cream
Laneige Bright Renew Original Cream

OCCASIONAL TREATMENTS

Hydrating Sheet Masks

Once in a while, I feel like I need an extra boost of moisture in my routine, so I'll reach for a hydrating mask in lieu of my usual serum. Bonus: most sheet masks provide a temporary brightening effect as well as making tired skin feel less hot and puffy!

> I LIKE:
> *My Beauty Diary Black Pearl Mask (Taiwanese)*
> *Leaders Insolution Coconut Gel Recovery Masks*
> *L'Herboflore Hyaluronic Acid Moisture Energy Biocellulose Mask (Taiwanese)*

Clay Mask

My skin is pretty well-behaved these days, but once in a while my T-zone turns into a nasty, oily mess. What to do? Apply a little mud mask!

> MY GO-TO CLAY MASK:
> *Queen Helene Mint Julep Mask (U.S. American)*
> This is my staple for drying up excess oil and temporarily shrinking enlarged pores.

Facial Oil

My skin gets very dehydrated and angry in the winter, and sometimes simple cream isn't enough. In those situations, I'll add a couple of drops of facial oil to my cream—that way, I get the benefits of the oil without making my face feel too greasy.

> MY FAVORITE:
> *Goodal Repair Plus Essential Oil*

Sleeping Pack

On days when my skin is feeling really dehydrated, or I want a little extra boost of glow, I'll apply a sleeping pack after my nighttime cream. This helps lock in moisture even more.

MY ALL-TIME FAVORITE:

TonyMoly Intense Care Dual Effect Sleeping Pack

It's very thick, which might not be everybody's cup of tea, but really does lock in the moisture. My skin always looks super-radiant after I use it.

Massage

Facial massage improves circulation and just feels good. It's sort of difficult to explain this step in words, but if you look up "gua sha" on the internet you'll find lots of information and tutorials. I do this on clean skin, maybe once every couple of weeks.

Mists

Facial mists can be super-refreshing, especially on hot, dry days. They're also useful if you wait a little bit too long between the "layers" of your skincare routine and want to top them off with moisture between steps.

I LIKE:

Missha's Time Revolution The First Treatment Essence Mist

The Skin House Aloe Water Mist

Acne Patches

I don't get too many severe breakouts these days, but once in a while, a monster zit will appear for no apparent reason. Instead of weeping and cursing the heavens, I apply a hydrocolloid acne patch. Hydrocolloid stickers react with the pus (ew) in your zit to draw it out, which helps them flatten and heal faster. Added bonus: having a physical barrier on your face keeps you from picking!

MY PREFERRED ACNE PATCH:

Nexcare Acne Absorbing Covers (U.S. American)

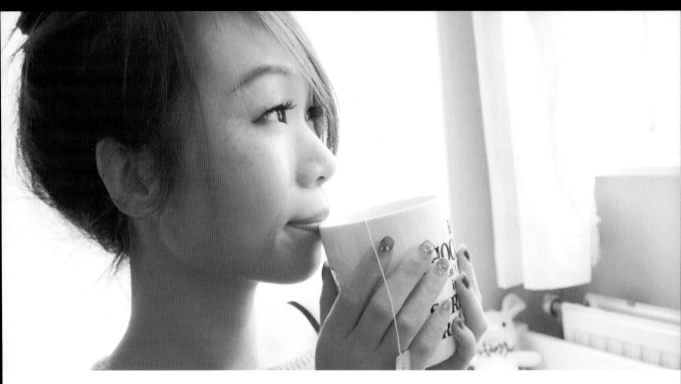

MEMORABLE DAYS

www.memorable-days.net

Elisa reviews a wide range of Korean skincare and makeup products from popular affordable brands such as Etude House, Innisfree, and Missha. She combines her passion for photography by taking gorgeous pictures of products and clear, color-accurate swatches for everything she reviews. Korean brand move very quickly when releasing new products, and if you want to stay up-to-date with new collections and product releases, her blog is a great resource!

SKIN TYPE
Combination/dry skin

SKIN CONCERNS
Dry and sometimes flaky cheek and mouth area, oily T-zone, dark spots, uneven skin tone, large pores

CLIMATE
Spring, cold, and windy in Amsterdam

HOW I GOT INTO K-BEAUTY
I started using Korean beauty products 5 years ago. The first product I tried was the Missha M Perfect Cover BB Cream, which is still very popular, even after so many years. I couldn't seem to find a good foundation shade for my Asian skin tone, which is why I decided to try Korean BB creams. Now I'm addicted to them and Korean products in general!

MORNING SKINCARE ROUTINE

1. Cleanse
Konjac Jelly Massage Cleansing Puff (Japanese)
In the morning, I clean my skin with the Konjac Jelly Massage Cleansing Puff and I splash my face five times with lukewarm water. Konjac sponges are made from plant fiber of konjac, grown in Japan. They are very gentle on the face and include ingredients that nourish and smooth the skin naturally. I can easily remove my face oil with it, leaving a soft and clean face afterwards.

2. Toner
Hada Labo Super Hyaluronic Acid Hydrating Face Lotion (Japanese)
This is one of my favorite products that I've been using for years. It contains a high percentage of hyaluronic acid which will moisturize your skin. I only need four drops for my entire face, I just dab it on and it instantly hydrates my skin and it helps to preserve its optimum moisture balance.

3. Ampoule
Missha Time Revolution Night Repair Science Activator Borabit Ampoule
I love to use this ampoule day and night. It energizes, brightens, and improves the elasticity of my skin. Besides that, it also has anti-aging benefits which is a plus for people in the mid-twenties like me.

4. Essence
Innisfree Green Tea Moisture Essence
Since I need more moisture for my dry skin, I'm using an additional essence. The texture of this essence is thicker than the previous two products, so that's why i'm using it afterwards.

5. Eye Serum
Dr. Jart+ V7 Eye serum
To brighten my eye area I'm using the V7 eye serum from Dr. Jart+. I love this serum since it sinks into my skin within seconds without leaving a heavy and sticky finish.

6. Sunscreen
Nuganic Customize Sun Block Fresh SPF50 PA+++
I love using Asian sunscreens since they have a high SPF, which I need to prevent getting more freckles on my face. It also leaves a moist finish that is not heavy or sticky, which is great for people with dry skin. It also contains anti-aging ingredients.

7. Cream
Paula's Choice Shine Stopper Matte Finish (U.S. American)
Sometimes I just prefer to have a matte finish, so I dab the shine-stopper from Paula's Choice on my T-zone and no shine will be visible afterwards. This is definitely one of my holy grails! I love the silky soft matte finish that it gives me and I will usually stay matte for at least five hours after application.

8. Lip Treatment
Vaseline Lip Therapy Original (U.S. American)
I can't live without this vaseline! It always feels that there is something missing if I don't apply Vaseline afterwards. It keeps my lips moist and it's scentless which I love.

EVENING SKINCARE ROUTINE

1. Makeup Removing Cleanser
Shu Uemura Porefinist Cleansing Oil (Japanese)
Using circular motions with my fingers, I massage and clean the makeup off of my face. It feels lightweight and fresh and since it contains cinnamon bark extract, it will target excess oil and controls my sebum.

2. Facial Cleanser
Hado Labo Gokujyun Face wash (Japanese)
I have been using this face wash for three years and I am still loving it. I am using this together with the Clarisonic MIA 2 to foam it up and to remove my makeup. It keeps my skin fresh and moist, without leaving a tight feeling afterwards. It does a very good job of removing heavy makeup, which is why I have been using this for years.

3. Eye Makeup Remover
L'Oréal Paris Dermo-Expertise Absolute Make-Up Remover Eye and Lip (French)
With a Q-tip I remove the remaining waterproof makeup off my eyes, mainly in the corners and tight-line area. The oil in this makeup remover erases everything thats waterproof in a second.

4. Cleansing Water
Innisfree Calming Cleansing Water
I'm always scared to have remaining makeup on my face, so that's why I put a bit of cleansing water on a cotton pad and go over my face and neck just once to make sure I catch any leftover makeup. This cleansing water is suitable for sensitive skin and is very gentle. It contains dandelion extracts and is full of glucocide and vitamins to smooth the skin. Because of this, it has a good pH level and my skin feels calm, moist, and refreshed afterwards.

5. Serum
Pure Vitamin C20 Serum
To lighten up my freckles and dark spots I use three drops of the vitamin C serum from OST. I feel a tingling sensation after and I normally will wait for twenty minutes to let it sink in, before I move on with the next step.

6. Toner
Missha Time Revolution The First Treatment Essence
Ever since I've been using this essence toner, my skin texture has improved and it gives my skin that hydration boost that I love. It made my skin soft, and reduced the dry flakes and redness on my face.

7. Ampoule
Missha Time Revolution Night Repair Science Activator Borabit Ampoule
I love to use the ampoule with the essence from Missha. Both products have improved the elasticity of my skin.

8. Essence
Innisfree Green Tea Moisture Essence

9. Eye Cream
Dr. Jart+ V7 Serum

10. Cream
Innisfree Green Tea Seed Cream
The Green Tea Seed Cream is enriched with green tea seeds which makes the skin moist. What I really love about this cream is that it absorbs quickly while leaving my skin soft and supple. I absolutely love the cooling effect and the scent of this cream too; it's so fresh!

11. Lip Treatment
Vaseline Lip Therapy Original

SPECIAL TREATMENTS

Wash-off Masks
Innisfree Volcanic Pore Clay Mask
Since I have a combination skin, it's important to treat certain parts differently. I use the Innisfree Volcanic Pore Clay Mask on my T-zone and chin area, which are the areas where my pores are more visible and where I tend to get more oily. It controls my oil really well.

Skinfood Rice Mask Wash Off
While leaving the volcanic pore clay mask on my T-zone, I use a rice mask wash off from Skinfood to moisture the rest of my face. I use this once a week.

Exfoliator
Cure Natural Aqua Gel (Japanese)
When I notice that I have dry flakes, I use this mild scrub to remove them. It's a great product for removing dead skin cells while leaving your skin moist.

Sheet Mask
My Beauty Diary Apple Polyphenol (Taiwanese)
Once a week, I use My Beauty Diary's Apple Polyphenol Sheet Mask to moisturize and brighten my face.

Spot Treatment
Ciracle Pimple Solution Pink Powder
When I notice that a pimple is coming up, I use the pink powder from Ciracle. This really is my holy grail! It hastens the healing process and it prevents acne scars.

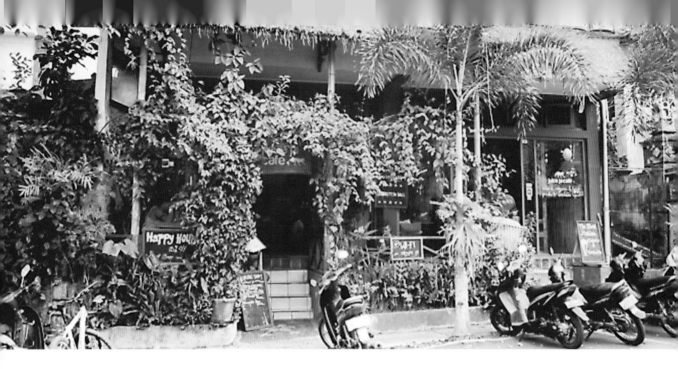

THE WANDERLUST PROJECT

www.thewanderlustproject.com

The Wanderlust Project is a travel, lifestyle, and Korean beauty blog. I live in Ho Chi Minh City, Vietnam, where the weather is hot and humid every single day. I ride a motorbike as my main form of transportation, so I'm worried about sun damage. I also have to deal with heavy pollution, dirt, and grime.

SKIN TYPE

I have combination skin with an oily T-zone. My skin is pretty normal everywhere else, although I did suffer from acne when I first moved to Vietnam.

SKIN CONCERNS

My major skin concerns are post-inflammatory hyperpigmentation, general evenness, and brightening of my skin tone.

HOW I DISCOVERED KOREAN COSMETICS

Before I moved to Vietnam, I lived in South Korea for two years. During that time, I fell in love with Korean cosmetics. I had pretty awful acne when I first moved to South Korea, but adopting a Korean skincare routine and using high quality, effective skincare products pretty much cleared up my acne. Now that I've introduced chemical exfoliants into my routine, I've achieved almost perfect skin!

MORNING SKINCARE ROUTINE

1. Cleanser
Su:m37 Miracle Rose Cleansing Stick
This varies daily, but this is my all-time favorite cleanser.

2. Acid Toner
Biologique Recherche P50 Lotion (French)
When I use the P50 Lotion, I wait twenty to thirty minutes before my next skincare step. If I'm in a rush, I'll either just use my vitamin C serum, or I'll skip this step completely.

3. Vitamin C
C21.5 Vitamin C Serum

4. Hydrating Toner
The Missha First Treatment Essence
This is my holy grail!

5. Moisturizer
Su:m37 Waterfull Gel Lotion
I'm currently rotating a few, but this one of my favorites. It's lightweight, and perfect for the hot, humid weather in Vietnam.

6. Sunscreen
Bioré UV Aqua Rich Watery Essence Sunscreen SPF 50+ PA++++ (Japanese)

EVENING SKINCARE ROUTINE

1. Makeup Removing Cleanser

Su:m37 Melting Cleansing Balm
This is my all time favorite!

2. Cleanser

Su:m37 Miracle Rose Cleansing Stick
Again, I love the Su:m37 Miracle Rose Cleansing Stick. I'm also testing out a bunch of different options like the Skinmiso Rice Foam Cleanser, the Hada Labo Anti-Aging Collagen cleanser, and the Klairs Rich Moist Foaming Cleanser.

3. Acid Toner/BHA/AHA Treatment

Biologique Recherche P50 Lotion (French)
COSRX BHA Blackhead Power Liquid
Mizon AHA 8% Peeling Serum
I rotate through these treatments depending on the day. I use each of these products to help with my large pores, my PIH, and general skin evenness and brightening. I apply one of these, and then wait twenty to thirty minutes before my next step.

4. Hydrating Toner

The Missha First Treatment Essence
I love the Missha First Treatment Essence, but I've also tried the Hera Cell Bio Essence, and the Hada Labo Lotion.

5. Serum

Hera Hyaluronic Ampoule
Right now, I'm focusing on hydrating and plumping my skin.

6. Moisturizer

HERA Aquabolic Emulsion
Su:m37 Time Energy Emulsion
Hada Labo Anti-Aging Milk (Japanese)
At night, I like to opt for something a bit more hydrating, so I reach for one of these three products.

7. Facial Oil

Su:m37 Fermented Argan Oil
I am beyond obsessed with this oil. Sadly, it's been discontinued, and I may have bought two of the last bottles!

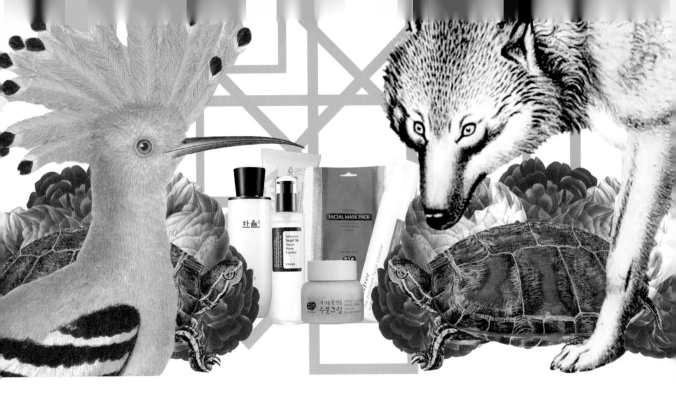

THE BEAUTY WOLF

www.thebeautywolf.com

I'm Coco Park, a beauty journalist, blogger, professional makeup artist, certified esthetician, and one of the authors of the book you're reading right now! My blog brings you only the best products I've discovered on my journey, roaming the plains of makeup and forging the rivers of skincare. I also illustrate my blog with one-of-a-kind artwork and collages.

SKIN TYPE
Normal to dry

SKIN CONCERNS
Sensitivity, reactivity, and acne-prone. I focus on relieving dryness, preventing further photoaging, refining, and restoring firmness

WHY I LOVE K-BEAUTY

The proof is in the pudding. I've totally transformed my skin. Before I discovered Korean products, my skin was plagued with redness, breakouts, and dryness. Now my skin is clear, healthy, and glowing. I couldn't be happier and I cannot shut up about it. I'll tell anyone who will listen about the virtues of K-beauty. So listen up: it's amazing and you need it in your life!

MORNING SKINCARE ROUTINE

1. Facial Cleanser

Innisfree The Minimum Facial Cleanser
Dr. Oracle The Snow Queen Enzyme Powder Wash
I start my morning routine with a low-pH facial cleanser, and like to rotate between these two.

2. First Treatment Essence

Missha Time Revolution First Treatment Essence
I will always reach for a first treatment essence. I once left it out of my routine for a month when I ran out, and never again. The difference is noticeable when I use it.

3. Hydrating Toner

Whamisa Organic Flowers Deep Rich Essence Toner
This water-free toner is everything. It smells like a garden in summertime and is full of hydrating, organic, skin-nutritious ingredients. Knowing I'm about to use this toner gets me happy to do my skincare routine in the morning.

4. Sheet Mask

Ideally, time permitting, I like to start my day with a sheet mask. I have several that I cycle through. My absolute favorites are:

Whamisa Organic Fruits & Tomato Fermented Hydrogel Facial Mask
This is a new holy grail and one of the best soothing, hydrating masks I've ever tried.

Whamisa Organic Sea Kelp Facial Sheet Mask

This is my special occasion mask, it's the champagne and caviar I treat my skin to. What makes this sheet mask different (aside from absolutely bursting with natural skin loving ingredients) is that the sheet is made from a piece of sea kelp, making you into the fanciest human kimbap of all time.

Klairs Rich Moist Soothing Mask

This is a little moisture bomb of a mask with a very soft, thick, cottony sheet. It also boasts a few of my favourite ingredients like natto gum and licorice root extract. At around $2 USD a mask, it's a great way to impart some moisture into the start of your day.

5. Serum

I alternate between these two, one week for one and then the next week for the other.

Su:m37° Secret Repair Concentrate

Always a favorite that I miss whenever I run out. I've taken to always having backups on hand.

COSRX Advanced Snail 96 Mucin Power Essence

Anyone that knows me knows I'm a huge fan of snails!

6. Emulsion

Hanyul Rice Essential Skin Emulsion

I love the feel of this on my skin and I love the look of it on my dresser. This has an insanely low number of acne triggers and is hydrating, yet light enough to not pill up under makeup or skincare.

7. Cream

Whamisa Organic Flowers Water Cream

This is another water-free treasure from Whamisa. I can't live without this stuff. It's perfect as is in the warmer months, but with my dry skin and the harsh winter climate I live in, I usually mix a few drops of maracuja or baobab oil in with this. If I could recommend just one cream to people starting out in K-beauty it would be this one. It's so wonderful!

8. Sunscreen
As someone who had skin cancer removed from the tops of my ears at a fairly young age, I am all about the sun protection now. Depending on the season, I use one of two sunscreens from Innisfree:

Innisfree Eco Safety Perfect Sunblock SPF50+ PA+++
This is my preferred sunscreen for cold winter weather.

Innisfree Eco Safety Aqua Perfect Sun Gel SPF50+ PA+++
This is a lighter weight sunscreen for warm and humid days.

9. Mist
Whamisa, the Organic Flowers Olive Leaf Mist
Whamisa Organic Flowers Damask Rose Petal Mist
I always carry around a mist for freshening up or for a little extra hydration. like to keep one in my bag and one in the fridge for extra refreshing home use.

EVENING SKINCARE ROUTINE

1. Makeup Removing Cleanser
Su:m37 Skin Saver Melting Cleansing Balm
First I start with an oil-based cleanser. Right now I'm head-over-heels in love with this cleansing balm. It's like heaven in a beautiful jar and it gently removes even the toughest makeup (including eye lash glue, which is the devil incarnate).

2. Facial Cleanser
Innisfree The Minimum Facial Cleanser for Sensitive Skin
I follow that up with this low-pH bubble cleanser.

3. First Treatment Essence

Missha Time Revolution First Treatment Essence

Just like my AM routine, this kickstarts my skin treatments.

4. pH Adjusting Toner

Mizon AHA & BHA Daily Clean Toner

Since I'm about to follow up with an acid, I like to get my skin down to the correct pH for it to work optimally.

5. Serum

Mizon AHA 8% Peeling Serum
OST Original Pure Vitamin C20 Serum

I use these to keep my skin properly exfoliated and bright.

6. Essence

Hanyul White Chrysanthemum Powder Serum

I've been in love with this serum since the first time I used it. It's worked like nothing else ever has to even out my skin tone.

7. Emulsion

Isoi Go Above And Beyond Lotion

This is a wonderfully light, yet hydrating emulsion with low acne and irritation triggers. I also love the smell of this lotion; it reminds me of a spring garden, which is very lovely to smell as you're settling into bed.

8. Cream

Depending on the season, I switch between two options.

> *Sulwhasoo Concentrated Ginseng Renewing Cream*
> In the harsh winter I love using this cream—it goes on like rich butter and makes my skin so very happy.

Whamisa Organic Flowers Water Cream
This is my trusty cream for warmer temperatures. I like to mix in a few drops of tamanu oil with it.

9. Sleeping Pack

Holika Holika Pig-collagen Jelly Pack
TonyMoly Pure Farm Pig Collagen Jelly Cream

I never sleep without some type of mask pack. I've been in the hospital and cracked up nurses who've watched me carefully applying my sleeping packs. For a while now, I've been a big fan of the pig collagen varieties. I alternate between these two—they both deliver great results and I can't say I prefer one over the other. As long as I have one of them, my mornings are met with plumper, hydrated, happy skin!

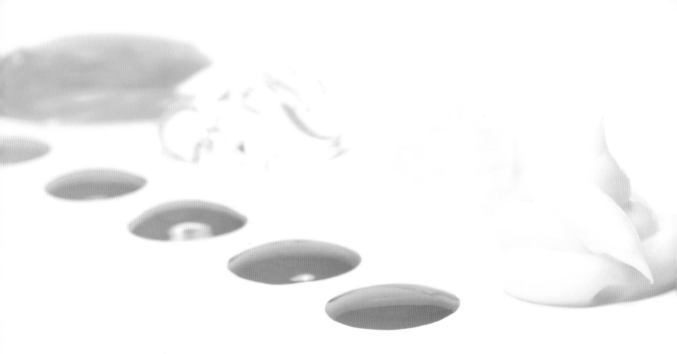

SKIN & TONICS

www.skinandtonics.com

My name is Kerry, and I am a writer, usability researcher, data analyst, designer, lifelong skincare enthusiast, and one of the authors of this book! My blog is dedicated to skincare guides and reviews of products from all over the world, with a special affinity toward Korean and Japanese products. I'm constantly altering my skincare routine, and it's important to me on a deeply personal level that my skincare be both highly effective *and* actively enjoyable. My love of luxury is matched only by my love of visible results.

SKIN TYPE
Normal to dry

SKIN CONCERNS
Prone to hormonally-triggered acne, post-inflammatory hyperpigmentation, occasional dehydration, mild sensitivity/reactivity. I am also devoted to line and wrinkle prevention.

WHAT I LOVE ABOUT KOREAN SKINCARE

Since I've adopted a Korean skincare approach, my skin health, clarity, luminosity, and resilience is the best it's ever been. But I what I love most is that the Korean beauty market seems to hold the same ideals about skincare as I do—the products tend to be just as interesting, luxurious, and fun as they are effective.

MORNING SKINCARE ROUTINE

1. Facial Cleanser

I wash with a low-pH cleanser in the AM to clear away any accumulated residue and sweat, in order to prepare a clean canvas for the day's skincare products.

> *Graymelin Moisture Cleanserum*
> This product is unlike any other cleanser I've used before. It is an extremely light, oilless, non-foaming, antioxidant cleanser that gently and thoroughly washes away any sweat or impurities that may have accumulated overnight. Its perfect 5.5 pH makes it ideal for all skin types. It cleanses away dirt and residue so effectively that I sometimes use it to remove makeup in the evening!

2. Acid (AHA/BHA) Toner

I follow up my second cleanse with an acid toner. Acid toners help refine skin texture by exfoliating the skin. By removing the dead skin cells, they also help increase the penetration of the products that follow. An acid toner can also help strengthen the moisture barrier by regulating the skin's pH, minimize excess sebum, reduce pore appearance, and prevent blackheads and blemishes.

> *COSRX AHA / BHA Clarifying Treatment Toner*
> I use this alcohol-free AHA/BHA liquid toner in the morning by swiping it over my face with a cotton pad.

3. BHA Treatment

Incorporating a BHA exfoliator into my routine has had one of the most dramatic impacts on my acne-prone skin. Combined with my other treatments, it's rare that a pimple ever fully forms, and the spots I do occasionally see don't stick around for long.

BHA Blackhead Power Liquid

I use this alcohol-free BHA liquid in the morning, which uses betaine salicylate as its BHA source as opposed to salcylic acid. It's gentler on my skin than many BHA formulas, while still being highly effective.

3. Hydrating Toner

For this step, I look for a product that's light and but loaded with enough humectants to provide sustained hydration for my skin.

Whamisa Organic Flowers Deep Rich Essence Toner

I love this alcohol-free toner for its light but richly-hydrating formula. Its fermented ingredients soothe facial redness, and it has the antioxidant concentration of a serum or essence. A few small drops is all I need to keep my skin hydrated all day long.

4. Essences, Serums, and Ampoules

This is the step that changes most often in my routine, and I'm frequently using more than one of these product types in order to target multiple concerns.

Hanyul White Chrysanthemum Powder Serum

This serum is packed with antioxidant-rich extracts, as well as lightening ingredients such as arbutin and kojic acid to keep my skin bright and help heal any post-acne red marks.

Banila Co The Black Pullulan Treatment Ampoule

This ampoule provides a solid dose of moisturizing yeast extracts, antioxidants, hydrating humectants, and an array of fatty-acid rich oils. It's soothing, light, moisturizing, and helps protect skin against free-radical damage.

5. Facial Oil

I like facial oils for their moisture-barrier-strengthening fatty acid content. During the day, I prefer a light yet nourishing oil that can deliver a boost of antioxidant and brighting ingredients.

Goodal Waterest Lasting Water Oil
This water oil strikes the perfect balance and contains humectant moisture in the form of glycerin, as well as an amazing blend of antioxidant and anti-inflammatory oils and extracts. It also contains brightening niacinamide and licorice root, and skin-barrier-friendly ceramide 3. It feels extremely light and non-greasy, yet the moisture it provides lasts for hours.

6. Cream

When I'm looking for a daytime cream, I make sure that it's occlusive enough to provide a protective seal for my previously applied hydrating ingredients, but without feeling sticky or interfering with the wear of my makeup. I also look for ingredients that are soothing, anti-inflammatory, promote skin health, and that will keep my complexion bright.

Goodal Moisture Barrier Cream
I use a thin layer of this mango seed butter based cream, which is amazingly occlusive while somehow managing not to feel heavy. It contains a slew of antioxidant-rich and anti-inflammatory plant extracts as well as niacinamide and ceramide 3. The finish for this cream is surprisingly smooth with no stickiness, making it great for wearing underneath makeup.

7. Sunscreen

I rotate through multiple favorites when it comes to sun protection. I look for sunscreen formulas that have strong, stable UVA protection in addition to UVB protection. I also need my sunscreen to wear well under makeup, and not feel too heavy.

Dr.G (Gowoonsesang) Brightening Up Sun Cream SPF PA+++
This is a great sunscreen formula that also contains anti-inflammatory and antioxidant-

rich plant extracts. It feels light, dries matte, and wears well under makeup.

EVENING SKINCARE ROUTINE

1. Point Makeup Remover

I wear a lot of eye makeup, and it's often waterproof, so I like to use a separate point makeup remover to thoroughly remove eyeliner, mascara, and brow gel without tugging. I really love dual-phase removers, which use a blend of water and silicone or oil to quickly and gently dissolve eye and lip makeup.

Innisfree Apple Juicy Eye & Lip Remover
This dual-phase remover works amazingly well, is extremely budget-friendly, doesn't sting my eyes, and smells like apple candy.

2. Makeup Removing Cleanser

When choosing a makeup removing cleanser for the first step of my double cleanse, I look for an oil-based cleanser that can gently dissolve even the most tenacious base makeup and sunscreen.

Banila Co. Clean-It Zero Cleansing Balm
This balm-textured cleanser turns to oil when applied to the skin. It dissolves makeup really well, and it smells like cherry blossoms. This is the makeup removing cleanser I reach for most often.

3. Facial Cleanser

In the evening, I follow up my makeup removal with a second cleanse to get rid of residual debris or traces of makeup. I look for a low-pH cleanser that thoroughly removes dirt without stripping my skin.

Su:m37 Miracle Rose Cleansing Stick
This slightly acidic solid cleanser smells amazing and creates a luxurious, low-foaming, silky lather that effectively cleanses my face without drying me out.

4. Acid Toner
I follow up my second cleanse with an acid toner in the evening, just as I do in the morning.

COSRX AHA / BHA Clarifying Treatment Toner

5. Actives & Treatments
After my acid toner, I apply products that contain my more heavy-duty actives such as prescription retinoids or AHA treatments. I don't use all of these every night—instead, I alternate treatments so I can get the most out of my products without irritating my skin.

Pocketderm Prescription (U.S. American)
Pocketderm is a U.S.-based online service in which an actual dermatologist provides a skincare consultation and prescription through their website or mobile app. I'm using an acne formula that contains Tretinoin, clindamycin, and azealic acid. I use this treatment 3 night a week.

Pure Vitamin C21.5 Advanced Serum
On nights when I'm not using my prescription treatment, I use this vitamin C serum to help keep my skin bright and to fade any post-acne discoloration I might have.

Papa Recipe White Flower Clear Up 8% AHA Gel
On the same nights when I use my vitamin C serum, I also like to use an AHA treatment. This chemical exfoliant prevents dullness and keeps my skin looking bright, even, and practically poreless.

6. Hydrating Toner
Just as I do in my morning routine, the product I use for this step should be light but provide plenty of humectant moisture.

Whamisa Organic Flowers Deep Rich Essence Toner

7. Essences, Serums, & Ampoules

In the evening, I look for rich ampoules and serums that are loaded with antioxidants, and contain ingredients that brighten skin or prevent acne flare-ups.

Graymelin Propolis 80 Energy Ampoule
Propolis is extremely high in antioxidants, provides nourishing moisture, and its antibacterial properties make it helpful for the treatment and prevention of acne breakouts. This particular ampoule contains a high percentage of propolis extract as well as hyaluronic acid, aloe, green tea, and ginseng extract.

Su:m37 Secret Repair Concentrate
This serum is easily the spend-iest item in my routine, but I love what it does for my skin. It's packed with fermented, antioxidant rich ingredients, barrier-strengthening ceramide 3, as well as skin-brightening niacinamide. It also feels and smells positively decadent.

8. Facial Oil

I top off my serums and ampoules with a little facial oil. In the evening I prefer an oil that feels light but will keep me moisturized through the night, and give me a big boost of nourishing antioxidants.

Goodal Repair Plus Essential Oil
I love this oil blend by Goodal, which is made with many of my favorite fatty acid and antioxidant-rich beauty oils including camellia, green tea seed, argan, and jojoba. It also includes fermented red yeast rice for an extra moisturizing boost that lasts into the following day. It's very nourishing, but feels light on my face.

9. Cream

At night, I want to seal in the moisture from my previous products as well as prevent water loss, which I'm particularly susceptible to after using my AHA or prescription retinoid treatments. I also like my creams to provide another dose of antioxidants.

Banila Co. Miss Flower & Mr. Honey Cream
This cream contains a generous dose of honey extract and yeast ferment, as well as a blend of some of my favorite fatty acid and antioxidant rich oils, including argan and evening primrose. It's extremely emollient and keeps my skin properly moisturized through the night, no matter how dry the air is in my bedroom.

SPECIAL TREATMENTS

Sleeping Pack

I use a sleeping pack at least three times a week to give my face additional treatment, nourishment, and moisture while I sleep. I look for moisturizing sleeping packs that will also give my skin an extra boost of antioxidants, and I consider the addition of brightening ingredients such as arbutin, licorice root, or niacinamide to be a huge plus. I always have several sleeping packs in rotation to choose from. Although my lineup changes frequently, I do have a couple of favorites that I find myself going back to again and again.

Isoi Bulgarian Rose Intensive Lifting Corset Mask
This mask starts off with a gelatin-like texture that spreads easily over the skin to create a nourishing layer of moisture that's readily absorbed and dries to a non-sticky finish. It smells delightfully like roses, and contains multiple antioxidant and anti-inflammatory extracts and oils, as well as skin brightening licorice root. Its interesting texture makes it a joy to apply, but even more joyous is the glowy, nourished complexion I wake up to when I've used this mask.

Sulwhasoo Overnight Vitalizing Mask
This is a rich, creamy sleeping mask that creates a wonderfully hydrating and emollient barrier over my skin. It's the mask I reach for if my skin is especially dry, when I'm recovering from a particularly nasty breakout, or if I've accidentally overdone it with a chemical exfoliant. In addition to infusing my face with moisture, it also contains barrier-boosting fatty acids, and a surge of antioxidant, anti-inflammatory, and brightening ingredients in the form of ginseng extract, green tea extract, licorice root, and arbutin. This mask makes my skin plump, smooth, and luminous.

Sheet Mask

I use a sheet mask during my evening routine two to three times per week. I look for sheet masks that will give me an immediate boost of hydration, and contain either healing, soothing, or skin-brightening ingredients.

Soo Ae Donkey Milk Skin Gel Mask Pack Whitening
This hydro gel mask is a powerhouse for dull or unevenly toned skin. It contains donkey milk, which is rich in amino acids, as well as antioxidant rich fruit and plant extracts. It also includes niacinamide, which is a great brightening and spot-lightening agent as well as an effective anti-acne and anti-aging ingredient.

Papa Recipe Bombee Honey Mask
This fiber mask is basically a honey grenade for your face. It's absolutely saturated with essence, which is full of moisturizing honey extract, healing propolis, a slew of antioxidants, and a little bit of brightening licorice root extract to round it all out. This mask has an immediate and dramatic plumping, calming, and moisturizing effect, and makes my skin look healthy and radiant.

Wash-off Mask

A wash-off mask a couple Saturdays per month provides me with additional exfoliating or purifying benefits.

Skinfood Black Sugar Strawberry Mask Wash Off
This is an all-time favorite—it's an sugar-based exfoliating mask that smells and looks like strawberry preserves. Because the sugar melts a bit when it comes in contact with wet skin, it's not as harsh as many physical exfoliators.

Too Cool for School Morocco Ghassoul Creamy Mousse Pack
Sometimes, especially during our humid summers, I crave a little purifying session with a clay mask. The mousse texture is fun and light. It leaves my skin smooth, my pores refreshed, and contains a little tea tree oil for some extra anti-acne power.

Spot Treatments

When I do have the occasional breakout, I reach for spot treatments that will speed up the healing process and minimize the severity.

Mizon Trouble Clinic Acence Blemish Out Pink Spot
This is a layered serum that contains calamine, AHA, and BHA ingredients to help dry the pimple and reduce inflammation. It drastically shrinks whiteheads overnight.

Ciracle Red Spot Cream
After I've successfully dried a spot, I apply this cream to the area for the next few nights. It contains zinc to help with inflammation, centella asiatica extract to reduce redness and prevent scarring, and tea tree oil to further treat the area and prevent the pimple from reanimating.

M

PERFECT COVER
B.B CREAM

SPF42 PA+++

NO.27

MISSHA M Perfect Cover B.B Cream
offers a novel skincare concept with
B.B cream, which lightens skin tone by
healing visible wrinkles and
blemishes with excellent skin-cover
ability, and prevents skin aging
through effective whitening and
anti-wrinkle properties.

MISSHA

PART 3
KOREAN MAKEUP

I still remember my first visit to a dedicated Korean cosmetics store—the phrase "like a kid in a candy store" comes to mind. It was probably as close to that experience as you can have as an adult. I was a die-hard North American and European luxury cosmetics consumer and hard to impress. Having worked as a makeup artist for years and as a student of esthetics in college, cosmetics has always been a big part of my life.

Even my first real job out of high school was working at a department store cosmetics counter. By the age of twenty, I had worked my way up to counter manager for a luxury brand before quitting to become a freelance makeup artist. I had been on both sides of the makeup aisle, so to speak, and pretty much thought I'd seen and knew it all. It had been a long time since the world of cosmetics retail excited me.

Upon walking into that first Korean cosmetics store, a cheery, brightly lit space lined with gorgeously packaged goodies, I was in awe. It was exhilarating! Each shelf was teaming with products calling to me to pick them up and explore. To my delight, not only was the packaging exciting, so were the formulations. I very quickly found items that not only matched the quality of my old holy-grail favorites; they surpassed them.

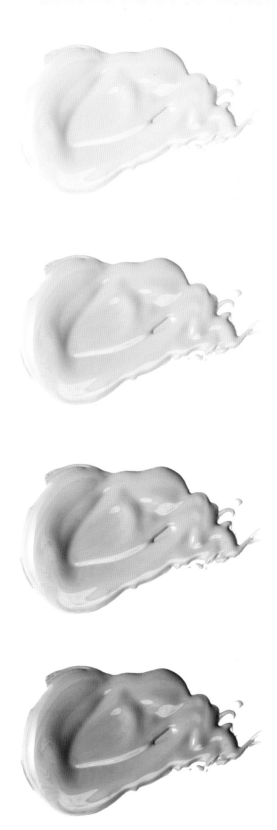

COMPLEXION

So let's start with that flaw-free canvas. If you're new to Korean beauty and don't yet have that dewy, flawless skin that's the hallmark of the Korean aesthetic, there are some products that can help you fake it till you make it.

BB CREAM

Unless you've just escaped a cult compound in the middle of the desert, I'm sure you've heard of BB cream. Depending on who you ask, the BB stands for beauty balm, blemish balm, or even *beblesh* balm. The origins of this cream can be traced all the way back to 1960s Germany, where a dermatologist formulated the balm to soothe and protect her patients' delicate new skin after facial peels and even surgery. Later, in the mid 80s, BB cream gained a huge following in Korea, thanks to actresses singing it's praises.

Today's formulations are marketed as a welcome replacement for heavy, cakey foundations. They usually contain skincare friendly ingredients, SPF, and have light reflecting properties that even out one's skin tone and blur blemishes. Since the BB creams of today are marketed mainly in the Asian market, sadly there are not a lot of shade options as of now. Most brands offer only two, perhaps three shade options on the light end of the spectrum that promise to oxidize within a few minutes to match your skin tone. That's all well and great if you are fair-skinned, but for those with darker skin, it can be frustrating finding a brand that you can rock. I'm hoping the huge surge in exports to other countries and the swelling popularity of Korean cosmetics will spur these companies on to produce a more generous offering of shades.

If you do fall within the very narrow shade spectrum, there are so many wonderful formulations for you to try. The majority of BB creams come in a traditional pump or squeeze tube, which you can apply with your fingers, a sponge, or a brush. I have a handful of such BB creams that I find myself purchasing again and again, recommending to friends, and using on photoshoots.

Missha M Perfect Cover BB Cream SPF 42 PA+++

The first is Missha M Perfect Cover BB Cream SPF 42 PA+++. This is Missha's most popular product; their website claims over 30 million have been sold worldwide. What I really appreciate about this product is its wider range of shades compared to other BBs. It may not sound like much compared to how many colors are available in other foundations, but with Missha's five shades options, we were able to match every girl at our photoshoot for this book. Missha's shade #31 Golden Honey is one of the darkest, if not *the* darkest, shade available in Korean BB creams. Conversely, #13 Milky Beige, is one of the fairest.

M Perfect Cover BB has medium-to-full, buildable coverage, and will easily cover minor flaws, even out skin tone, and help conceal under-eye discoloration. It also contains ingredients that are skin friendly, such as jojoba oil, rosemary extract, algae extract, caviar extract, and ceramides.

Dr. G Gowoonsesang Brightening Balm

If you want to reach back to the early origins of BB creams, there's Dr. G Gowoonsesang Brightening Balm. According to Gowoonsesang, the company was established by a team of medical skin professionals, including eight doctors, forty-three dermatologists, 114 nurses and 110 medical estheticians. This BB cream truly pays tribute to its doctor developed roots with a focus on skincare ingredients that brighten and even skin tone. However, I would only recommend this BB cream for cool, fair skin. It can read a little gray on warmer and darker tones. That said, it is *excellent* for addressing uneven skin tone and removing redness with its light, concealer-like coverage. It also does a bang-up job controlling oil and leaves a very natural matte finish as it melts into the skin. It's a must try for pale, cool-toned complexions seeking to balance out ruddiness!

Lioele Triple The Solution BB Cream

Another top pick is Lioele Triple The Solution BB Cream. This is one of the fuller coverage BB creams I've tried. I'd say it's more akin to a foundation in terms of coverage, but unlike a foundation, this covers without being cakey. Yogurt powder and licorice root extract are two of the notable ingredients in this formulation, along with an SPF rating of 30 PA++. It applies extremely smoothly and creamy.

Another thing that makes this high-coverage BB stand apart from foundations is that it doesn't cling to dry patches or settle into fine lines. The major drawback is that it's only available in a single shade, so this is going to work for only a very limited selection of people. It does oxidize, brighten, and then adjust to your color, but that's only if you fall within the narrow fair-to-medium toned family.

Innisfree Forest for Men Handsome BB SPF30 PA++

There are also BB creams marketed to men. They're billed more as a sunblock/moisturizer/skin treatment with some color correction, while avoiding the label "makeup." Spending an estimated $900 million a year on skincare and cosmetics, men in Korea are just as concerned about their skin as women.

There are several popular men's BB creams, and I actually have a favorite. My husband, who is a professional model, uses Innisfree Forest For Men Handsome BB SPF30 PA++ when he's on set or on the runway. Forest For Men BB has a lighter, more watery texture than any of the BB creams I use, and has a much more natural finish. It also works very, very well for oily skin. I say screw gender lines, if you're a female and

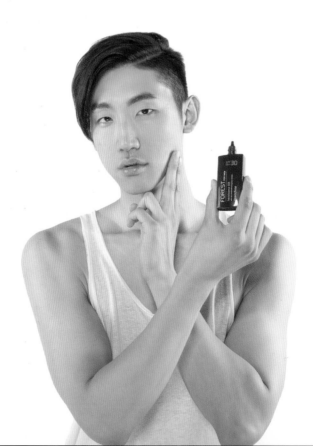

you think that formula sounds appealing to you, or a male who wants a thicker, more dewy formula found in women's BB creams, go for it!

Dr Jart+ Premium Beauty Balm SPF 45

Lastly, my other favorite BB tube is Dr Jart+ Premium Beauty Balm SPF 45. This BB is very similar to the Lioele cream in terms of wear and feel, but offers slightly less coverage. What it really has going for it is that it's very easy to purchase across the world since it's available at Sephora. It also has a leg up on the Lioele BB in the sense that Dr Jart is at least available in two shades: light to medium, and medium to deep. The tube is very sturdy, coated in a hard plastic, it travels well without fear of puncture.

CC CREAM

As if BB cream wasn't enough, there's also CC cream (and DD, EE, etc. cream but those are few and far between and not really worth getting into). CC cream is a branch of the BB cream/foundation family tree. CC usually stands for Color Correcting, and in that case, is designed to be used as color-correcting primer used under your BB cream. Promising to keep ruddiness and dull skin at bay, some formulas have enough coverage to even out skin tone and be worn alone.

Banila Co. It Radiant CC Cream SPF30 PA++

Banila Co. It Radiant CC Cream SPF30 PA++ is probably the most popular CC cream in the Korean beauty blogger world. With an herbal water complex, micro powders, and brightening capsules, this product lightens and brightens. So much so that I would only recommend this to fair-skinned people. Many CC creams are only available in a single shade. Therein lies the problem with a lot of traditional Korean CC creams: because of the trend of wearing foundation/BB cream a few shades lighter than your actual skin tone, these creams are incredibly whitening. Unless you are on the fairest end of the spectrum, many Korean CC creams are going to give you major "ghost face."

TonyMoly Pure Aura Luminous CC Cream

TonyMoly Pure Aura Luminous CC Cream does a good job providing a soft luminous finish that could be substituted for a BB cream if you don't have a lot of imperfections that need covering. This formula has the aforementioned micro capsules that break to reveal a bright, neutral beige color, housed inside an upright plastic tube with a pump, but again, only the very fair will benefit.

Borntree Bloom Mineral Avenue Ampoule CC SPF25 PA++

There's even an ampoule-style CC. Borntree Bloom Mineral Avenue Ampoule CC SPF25 PA++ comes in a glass jar with a dropper-style applicator, just like you'd find in an ampoule. It promises to moisturize and treat skin, as well as provide light coverage of imperfections. It's very shimmery and glowy upon application. I actually quite like this CC, and would love to see more ampoule-style CC's on the market!

Hera CC Cream Complete Care Cream SPF35/PA++

Now, for my absolutely favorite CC cream, the Hera CC Cream Complete Care Cream SPF35/PA++. Unlike the first two I mentioned, this one comes in two shades instead of the single shade. I still wouldn't recommend it for very tan or dark skin, but I'm happy there's at least the two options available. There is 01 Pink Beige, for cool pink undertones, and 02 Natural Beige for light to medium beige undertones. This cream blends smoothly, and gives an instant incandescent glow. While it's very moisturizing, it's loved by both oilier and drier skin types. It can very easily be worn both under and in place of a BB cream. Hera is the priciest CC cream, but I find it's also the very best, a pleasure to use, and worth the money if you're going to give one a try.

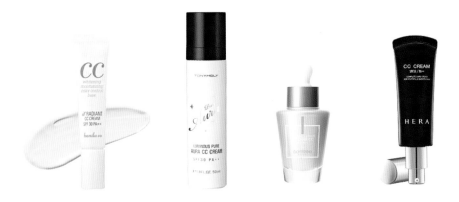

160

CUSHION COMPACTS

In addition to the conventional tube packaging for CCs and BBs, there's also the now ubiquitous cushion compact. It features a chubby compact that opens up to reveal a sponge soaked in BB cream that you apply with a provided silicone puff. The silicon pad gives an airbrushed finish when used with a light stamping or patting motion.

Some people were concerned that a sponge might not be sanitary with multiple uses, so now there are metal cushions available that dispense a squirt of BB when you depress the pan with the provided round sponge. In the case of CC creams, there are compacts much like the metal BBs, but with plastic pans that offer up a single squirt of product with each touch. For ease of use, portability, and flawless application I personally love BB cushions and their many ever-changing manifestations.

It's important to note that when using a cushion BB, you must hold the sponge flat in your fingers, and then stamp or pat on the foundation with a light touch. If you bend the applicator or press too hard, two things will happen: (1) the BB will not have that lovely airbrushed look that we usually get from the cushion, and (2) eventually, your sponge will split and tear. A bonus to the prescribed cushion-compact method is that you don't have to worry about buffing, blending, or getting a streaky application with your BB cushion.

This product is great for beginners and pros alike! I have tried so many different cushions for the purpose of blog reviews, and each time I thought it couldn't get any better I found more and more must tries.

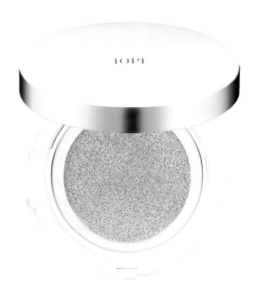

Iope Air Cushion

The Iope Air Cushion is a very popular version that I really love. Iope would be akin to a brand like Lancome in terms of pricing and prestige in Korea. It's on the higher end of the pricing spectrum, but is truly a great option. It comes in a couple of different finishes, natural (medium coverage) and cover (medium to full coverage). Sadly, as with most BB creams, there are only three shades available.

Iope brought the first BB cushion to market in 2008, and they have dominated the market ever since. With a formula that includes plant peptides, mineral water, and various vitamins, Iope boasts sales that average about one unit sold every four seconds. With a revenue of 200 million dollars in 2014, Iope has the number-one Korean market share for foundation products. Iope's parent company, Amore Pacific (which owns many major Korean brands), claims that one out of every 2.4 women between the ages of twenty and sixty-nine used Iope's Air Cushion.

And if you're wondering, yes, it really is that good! I find myself going back to it time and time again. Never cakey, never falling into fine lines, and with a broad spectrum SPF 50, it's an excellent choice. I've known both oily skin types and dry skin types to like this one, so it's suitable for just about anyone. It normally retails somewhere around $40–$45 , and usually comes with a free refill for each compact.

Innisfree Ampoule Intense Cushion

Another BB cushion I've not only enjoyed, but also repurchased, is the Innisfree Ampoule Intense Cushion. Like Iope, it's available only in three shade selections, but it is approximately $10 cheaper. It's billed as being for the drier months of the year, but I think anyone with normal to dry skin would enjoy this at any given time. Containing green tea leaf extract, green tea seed oil, sodium hyaluronate, orchid, and niacinamide, and scoring exceedingly low on the acne trigger scale, this cushion provides a glowing, dewy finish without being greasy.

My only complaint about this cushion is that it only has an SPF of 34, but you shouldn't be getting your only sun protection from your BB cream anyway, so that isn't much of a drawback.

Innisfree Water Glow Cushion

A sister product in the Innisfree line, the Water Glow Cushion, has a higher SPF of 50. It also boasts green tea extract, an excellent moisturizer, antioxidant, emollient, and astringent as its first ingredient. This product, as its name indicates, gives a watery, glowing finish. The cushion's ingredients will give your skin moisture without any kind of heaviness or stickiness. Like the others, it also scores very low on acne triggers, so anyone battling breakouts has little to worry about with this product.

The Missha M Magic Cushion

All of the cushions I've talked about so far have dewy finishes, but if you're looking for something a little different, Missha has a great option for you. The Missha M Magic Cushion has a very unique finish that strikes the perfect balance between matte and dewy. Housed in substantial packaging that includes a mirror, this cushion feels very high end. This BB pats onto the skin slightly orange, but oxidizes into a nice warm shade. The coverage is medium and is applied best with a light touch. Since the formula skews toward matte, it's not as forgiving to a heavy hand as an ultra dewy finish would be. The Missha cushion also has a very pleasant, clean, scent that is very fresh and floral.

One of my favorite things about this BB besides the finish is how powdery soft your skin feels after application. You'll have a hard time stopping yourself from touching your face; I know I did. With ingredients like baobab fruit extract, witch hazel, bamboo water, niacinamide, xylitol, and cactus flower extract, this BB is very friendly to oily skin and has very low acne trigger content. The driest of skins might want to do with a more emollient BB, but I'm normal to dry and I really like it. It's the perfect cushion for all the matte looks that are gaining in popularity.

VOLUMER & HIGHLIGHTERS

Although BB cushions are my preferred method of application, there are times when I do need a traditional BB tube. One of those times is when I'm using volumer-type products. What is a volumer? Well, if you've ever watched any Korean television shows, movies, or music videos, you might have noticed that the stars have this ethereal, youthful, dewy, glowing skin. It's mesmerizing and almost otherworldly. Yes, that is in large part thanks to their skincare, but you can also achieve this look with a volumer! It's a clear, or slightly iridescent liquid or cream that you can mix in a 1:3 ratio with your favorite BB cream, or directly add it to areas that you would normally apply highlight to, such as the tops of the cheeks, cupid's bow, forehead, and nose bridge. It's called a volumer because it adds a dewy "volume" to your face.

I know that glowing skin flies in the face of the matte, powdered-down, North American aesthetic that's been popular for years, but I think it's such a beautiful look. As you age, the first thing you notice is that your glow disappears, so adding a volumer can help your skin look more youthful.

Volumers can also be used on any skin color, so even if you are shaded out of the BB cream market, you can still use a volumer-type product with your foundation of choice. Anyone can have that enviable dewy look, from the very lightest to the very darkest skins.

Etude House Nymph Aura Volumer

My favorite is the original Etude House Nymph Aura Volumer, which comes in two options, a transparent and a pinky-iridescent shade. They also contain argan and avocado oil.

VDL Lumilayer Primer

If you want a more subtle glow, another favorite of mine is the VDL Lumilayer Primer. Although billed as a primer, which you can absolutely use it as, it can also be mixed with your BB or foundation at a 1:1 ratio. The Lumilayer Primer is iridescent, reflecting a gorgeous violet, red, and blue color that presents as a clear reflective surface on the skin.

According to their ad copy "VDL's Lumilayer Primer contains a Violet Lightflects pigment which evens out the skin tone while creating a clear, radiant and healthy skin for the next step of makeup. This primer is also creates a 3-dimensional face line by reflecting light from all angles of the face. I also appreciate that it has almost no acne triggers, so it's very friendly to those prone to breakouts.

Beauty Oil or Essence as Volumer

Another trick for anyone of any skin tone trying to get that dewy glow is to mix a few drops of your favorite beauty oil (such as argan, or maracuja) with your foundation. If you'd still like to have soft-lit skin with a little extra oomph, but are going for a more matte look, swap out the oil for your skincare treatment essence of choice. I always like to try to find ways for my products to pull double duty, and marrying your skincare to your makeup is always an added bonus.

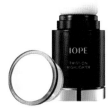

Iope Twist-On Highlighter

Iope Twist-On Highlighter delivers a iridescent highlighter powder with one twist of the package. Twist the product to reveal a cushy, cotton-y applicator, then click again for the highlighter. Each click measures out the perfect amount of product to tap onto your face. A powder highlighter like this works especially well if you'd like to go with the more subtle dewy look that's cropping up on the streets of Korea.

For that look, apply your normal dewy-but-not-overly-glossy BB cream, such as Missha's M Magic Cushion, which is a more matte finish BB cushion. You could possibly even go over it with a mattifying powder such as Innisfree No Sebum Mineral Pact (which is my very favorite), then apply the highlighter on the "C zones" which are around the orbital bone. You can also apply across the forehead and tops of the cheeks.

Basically, apply it anywhere you want the illusion of volume, since a loss of volume is a visual signifier of aging. Those areas are some of the first to show a depletion of the youthful fat in faces, and where injectable fillers are usually targeted. Trust me, it's the saddest I've ever been over losing fat.

Nature Republic Botanical Highlighter Stick

Another highlighting product that stands out to me is the Nature Republic Botanical Highlighter Stick. I was on set with two other makeup artists and brought this product along with me, and as the day went on, both of them reached for it continuously. It ended up on every model we handled that day, which was six girls ranging from dark mocha to vanilla skin tones.

This creamy, twist-up, stick highlighter comes housed in a plastic bullet tube. It's available in two shades, 01 Shine Pink and 02 Shine Gold. The silvery sheen in Shine Pink can read a bit ashy on very dark skin, but Shine Gold makes for a wonderful highlight on just about any skin color. Fairer skins will enjoy both Shine Pink and Shine Gold and can choose either depending on what direction they'd like to go in with their makeup. Shine Pink is good for sweet, cotton-candy-pink looks, and Shine Gold lends itself well for golden goddess looks. We especially liked Shine Gold with bold orange lips; it was the perfect shimmery complement to a warm citrus look.

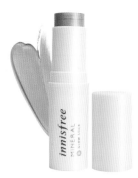

Innisfree Mineral Glow Stick

One more handy highlighter stick I like is the Innisfree Mineral Glow Stick. This highlighter is a lot more subtle than the Nature Republic Botanical Highlighter Stick. It comes in just a single shade and delivers a beautiful sheen. It looks darker and more bronze in the tube than it does on the skin, where it reads as a perfect, peachy shine. It has a fine microshimmer, so it's never chunky and very much suitable for daytime wear. It's also surprisingly tenacious and lasts on me for hours.

Innisfree Mineral Moisture Fitting Base

If you're looking for a liquid highlighter, wow, I don't even know where to begin, there are so many options! We've already touched on the Nymph Aura Volumer and the VDL's Lumilayer Primer, which are certainly a good option as a stand-alone highlighters. There's also Innisfree's Mineral Moisture Fitting Base, which is billed as a three-in-one shimmery primer, lotion, and cream, but could certainly be used as a highlighter alone. It contains ingredients such as shea butter, abalone pearl mineral, prickly pear, citrus, camellia, and orchid, which makes me feel like a fancy nature princess when I use it.

When buffed out as a primer, it leaves behind a subtle sparkle, but when used in concentration as a highlighter, it leaves behind a still subtle, but more obvious iridescent red-pink incandescence.

Innisfree Smart Make Up Blender (Shimmer)

If the "moisture" part of Mineral Moisture Fitting Base isn't right for your oily skin, worry not, Innisfree has an almost identical product called Smart Make Up Blender that will work better with oily-to-combination skins. If you have trouble with excess sebum in the T zones, this one comes without the heavy duty moisturizers.

It also has a tiny price tag because it comes in a tiny tube. Compared to the Mineral Moisture Fitting Base which is around $18 USD at 40ml, Innisfree Smart Make Up Blender (Shimmer) weighs in at a featherweight 15ml and retails for about $8. Innisfree offers Smart Make Up Blender in four options: shimmer, cover, moisture, and long lasting.

Billed as being a primer of sorts that can be mixed in a ratio of 1:2 with your foundation or BB, once again this can pull double duty as a highlighter. This settles into pretty much the same color as the Mineral Moisture Fitting Base. I'm looking at both of them on the back of my hand right now and I would say the Smart Make Up Blender (Shimmer) is ever-so-slightly less pink and has a smidge more peach in its iridescence. If they weren't side by side you probably wouldn't notice much difference.

Innisfree Smart Make Up Blender (Shimmer) also contains the amazing nature-derived ingredients that are the hallmark of the Innisfree brand. Products of note, are the amethyst powder, coral powder, pearl powder (which explains that ethereal shine), along with green tea leaf extract, citrus peel extract, and sodium hyaluronate.

Finally, here's a little pro tip for highlighters: apply them to your collar bones, tops of shoulders, and down your arms, for an unexpected sexy-all-over luminosity. It's a little detail that not everyone might think of, that makeup artists sometimes employ during runway shows and photoshoots. Overall, there a lot of great options—the world of highlighters is your oyster; time to pick your pearl!

CONCEALER

I can't talk about complexion makeup and not *cover* concealers (haaa!). My only grievance with Korean concealers is the same annoyance I have with the BB and CC creams, the lack of shade selections. There are just as few, if not less, color options for concealers marketed in Korea. So keep that in mind as I talk about my favorites, because sadly, they made them only for fair-to-medium skin tones. However, if you do fit in this small slice, be prepared to find your next crown jewel.

I am completely enamored with Korean concealers. With North American or European concealers I was always in a constant battle with it seeping into fine lines, highlighting dry patches, and giving cakey coverage. I had tried just about every major brand and formula and I was never happy. I've since found concealers from Korean companies that I've fallen head-over-heels for.

Skinfood Salmon Darkcircle Concealer Cream

My top pick is definitely Skinfood Salmon Darkcircle Concealer Cream. This rich, creamy concealer never ever settles into my fine lines and completely covers my dark circles, no matter how much I've aggravated them with lack of sleep. With its buttery consistency, this concealer is perfect for those with mature and/or dry skin.

Available in only two shades, this would be best for fair to very-light medium skin. It brightens, conceals, corrects, all without getting cakey or tacky. I would use this strictly under or around the eyes; for blemishes I would recommend a more viscous formula, such as Clio Kill Cover Pro Artist Liquid Concealer.

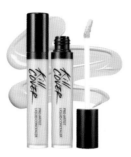

Clio Kill Cover Pro Artist Liquid Concealer
Clio's Kill Cover concealer is available in five shades to match a wider variety of skin tones, has a matte finish, and is very high coverage.

3 Concept Eyes Full Cover Concealer
3 Concept Eyes Full Cover Concealer is another high coverage concealer, but is available in just two shades. This concealer is liquid, but creamy, so I like to use it on lips to cover natural pigment when doing a dramatic gradient lip.

Missha The Style Under Eye Brightener
I have one more selection that I love to recommend to people who want to cover up dark circles, but hate concealer. I've called Missha The Style Under Eye Brightener my "anti-concealer" before, as it does everything you want a concealer to do without the concealer look. Available in only two shades, it uses light reflective properties to diffuse the look of discoloration under the eye. It's very subtle but very, very effective. I always look refreshed, bright-eyed, and ready for the day after using this product. The fact that it retails for $5 makes it a must-try for anyone that fits within it's narrow shade range.

PRIMER

To wrap up all things complexion, I'm going to take you back to the very first step: a primer. In Korean makeup, primer doesn't always mean a base coat on your skin that helps makeup adhere to it; it can also mean a pre makeup skin prep. A lot of primers would be better suited being called "preppers." With skin-beneficial ingredients, light diffusers, and sometimes, emollients, these primers are a great way to ready your face for the masterpiece you're about to apply to it.

The Face Shop Mango Seed Glow Date Prep Butter

One such "prepper" is The Face Shop Mango Seed Glow Date Prep Butter. I'm so glad I discovered this product, which was introduced to me by Mariella at The Face Shop's Montreal location (who by the way, was one of the most helpful, professional people I've ever encountered on a sales floor—shout out to Mariella for all of her help!).

I went in looking for something to prime my dry winter skin to receive makeup and came out with a must-have. This creamy primer helps makeup adhere to the skin by providing a smooth, moisturized base. It has a delicious, yummy smell, and provides a beautiful, moist glow for dry-to-normal skin types. I brought this primer with me on set and we used it on all the girls who were getting a dewy look. Every one of them loved it and asked me about the product afterwards.

It comes in a substantial jar and has a spatula included in the packaging so you needn't contaminate your product with germy fingers. This primer/prep would probably not be suitable for oily skins, as they might find the cream texture to be a bit much, but if your skin is dry or normal, you should really check this stuff out!

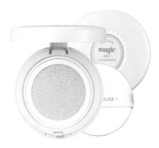

Etude House Mineral Magic Any Cushion

There are also primers aimed at correcting color. My top pick is Etude House Mineral Magic Any Cushion. Yes, this primer has the same delivery system as the BB cushions in their line, and it's wonderful! It comes in three color-correcting shades: mint for combating redness, pink to liven up pale complexions, and peach to brighten any dullness in tanned skin.

These primers go on extremely light and work with just about any skin type. I sometimes use the pink version of this to create a soft, pretty sunset look, which I'll demonstrate later.

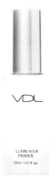

VDL Lumilayer Primer

I talked about how much I loved the VDL Lumilayer Primer in the Volumer and Highlighters section. I also really love it when used as a stand-alone primer. The Lumilayer Primer leaves a soft, diffused shimmer on your face without being overpowering and without feeling heavy or greasy. It's exceedingly lightweight, and therefore, oily and combination skins looking for a little extra something would enjoy this primer.

Innisfree No Sebum Mineral Primer

For those with oily skin who are looking for something to help soak up excess sebum and soften the look of open pores, Innisfree No Sebum Mineral Primer might be just the thing you're looking for. This primer removes shine, smooths skin, and leaves you with a matte complexion instantly.

For a longer-lasting matte finish you could follow it up with a sebum control powder. I like the Innisfree No Sebum Mineral Pact which is a no-frills workhorse of a powder that really goes the distance.

Peripera Oil Capture Pact

I also love the Peripera Oil Capture Pact, which comes in an adorable compact that keeps the puff separated from the product, much like a cushion compact. It has a mirror inside the pact that's great for touchups on the go.

Dr. Jart+ Pore Refine Recover Primer

Another, higher-end option for oily skins looking for a primer is Dr. Jart+ Pore Refine Recover Primer. If you're not a fan of talc in your products, then this would be a great option for you as it's completely talc free. It's long lasting, and does wonders for assisting your chosen BB cream or foundation to overcome destructive oil to perform the way it should.

Etude House's Proof 10 Eye Primer

Another type of primer that's just as, if not more, important is your eyeshadow primer. To keep your shadow's color true and long-wearing, a good primer is essential. One of my absolute favorite Korean cosmetics products of all time is Etude House's Proof 10 Eye Primer. I used to be devoted to Urban Decay's Primer Potion until I discovered this product. The Proof 10 Eye Primer is a quarter of the price of Urban Decay's primer, and performs even better in my experience. This is hands-down the only primer I reach for whether on set or at home.

It comes in a small bottle with a doe foot applicator wand, and a few swipes blended onto your eyelid is all you need to carry you through the day and into the night. This primer helps my shadow apply so much more vibrantly than it would sans primer, which is something that's very important when it comes to many Korean eyeshadows.

Eyeshadows have come a long way since I started exploring Korean cosmetics, but they are still less pigmented than North American or European formulations.

COLOR & POINT MAKEUP

Since skincare and complexion makeup is the main focus in Korean looks, a lot of the point makeup is very subtle and not heavily pigmented. There are some notable brands that do focus on bold color (VDL, 3 Concept Eyes) but for the most part, eyeshadows and blushes are a softer wash compared to, say, a NARS or MAC offering, but the formulas are wonderful and very interesting.

BLUSH

Blushes from Korean lines have recently received the same treatment that BB creams did: there are now many available in cushion form, and they're some of my top picks.

Iope Cushion Blusher

Iope Cushion Blusher comes in the same (but smaller) packaging as its BB Cushion sister. The application is a dream; it's almost impossible to mess up. Simply press the cushion with the provided silicone sponge and then pat onto your cheeks.

The blush itself is a creamy, sheer liquid that imparts a translucent dewy wash of color onto the cheeks, so you don't have to worry about going overboard and getting a severe 1980s streak of blush. This blush's color can be built somewhat, but for the most part, it is a very sheer product that's best suited to natural looks.

It's a great blush, but it's only available in two shades, sherbet peach and rose pink. Once again, I love the cushion packaging for its portability and ease of touch-ups.

PeriPera Ah Much Cushion Blusher

A slight variation on the cushion blusher compact is the PeriPera Ah Much Cushion Blusher. What makes this one different is that it's a tube with the cushion on the end. This cushion itself is also a bit different from the others. The typical cushion is a porous sponge-type material; this one is more like a soft, flocked, material—almost like a firm sponge coated with a soft velour-feeling texture.

To use it, you squeeze the tube and it delivers the blush to the cushion. From there, you tap it onto your cheeks straight from the applicator. It gives the same wonderful, soft wash of color as the cushion compact blush, but this one is even more portable and easy to apply, as it eliminates the need for the middle man: the sponge. It's a completely self-contained delivery system, so it's very easy to slip into your bag on the go. That's practically unheard of when it comes to blush.

PeriPera Ah Much Cushion Blusher is available in five shades, which is a more generous shade selection than the Iope Cushion Blusher. They are mostly pastel-type shades, so if you're looking for something crazy pigmented, this isn't the blush for you. However if you're looking for a dewy-sheer color wash, check out Sweet Pink, Oh! Blissful Coral, Yay! Happy Orange, Oh! Heart Fluttering Pink, and Haha! Crisp Lavender. Ranging from a warm beige pink, true coral, bright orange, and a fun, bubblegum-pink, one of these is sure to be just what you're looking for.

The Face Shop Lovely Me: Ex Pastel Cushion Blusher

If you're longing for something super-matte, sweet, and innocent, try The Face Shop Lovely Me: Ex Pastel Cushion Blusher. Now, this is not a cushion blusher like the ones we spoke about before. This is a traditional powder cake and puff blusher. The "cushion" in the name is referring to how cushiony-soft the puff is.

The blush shades are all very pastel as the name tells you; it's also very soft toned, like a baby's flush. These blushes can read as chalky on darker skin, so it's best to use these if your skin is fair-to-medium. It is available in five shades: 01 Rose Cushion, 02 Coral Cushion, 03 Plum Cushion, 04 Pink Cushion, and 05 Peach Cushion.

Although this current version is a rerelease and is in different packaging, the first releases were actually one of my first Korean cosmetic purchases. I got them from my first visit to The Face Shop in Pallisades Park, New Jersey. I ended up purchasing every color. They're so economical that I ended up buying every color in this updated version as well!

The Face Shop Lovely Me: Ex You & Face Blusher

The Face Shop also carries an equally cheap (in price, not quality!) blusher: Lovely Me:Ex You & Face Blusher. They come in a mix of matte and shimmer finishes and the line even includes a bronzer, contour shade, and two highlighter shades.

Choose from 01 Pink Glow, 02 Gold Glow, 03 Purple Fantasy, 04 Baby Pink, 05 Pink Affair, 06 Fuzzy Peach, 07 Pink Peach, 08 Orange Syrup, 09 Cinnamon Dream, and 10 Sandy Brown.

The Face Shop Soft Cream Blusher

I can't talk about The Face Shop blushes without including their Soft Cream Blusher. The Face Shop Soft Cream Blusher comes in only two shades, 01 Pink and 02 Coral, but they're both lovely. 01 Pink is a cool-toned, blue-based, bubblegum pink that can be buffed out into a very striking but natural flush on fairer skins. 02 Coral is a true traditional coral that lends itself a little better to more tanned skins, but could also work for fair skin if it's applied with a light touch.

These blushes give bold color without being overpowering and wear really well throughout the day.

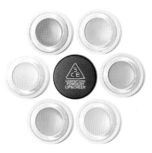

3 Concept Eyes Color Pots

Speaking of bold color, 3 Concept Eyes is always a brand when that's what you're looking for. They have several options for blush in their lineup, from pots, to powder, to cream. Their pots are meant to serve three functions, but I find that they perform best as blushes, although in a pinch, they could work on the eyes and lips. I've tried them that way before and while the results are very pretty, as an eyeshadow and lip color, there are much better wearing options out there. However, the color pots are great little blushers that travel well since they're in a pot and can be applied with your fingers.

3 Concept Eyes Powdery Lip & Cheek

3 Concept Eyes Powdery Lip & Cheek are available in five bright, cheery colors. Tibet Orange is a true bright orange—it's a bold choice and looks great with summery orange looks. Lingogo Hoho (yes, that's really what it's called) is a tomato red that errs on the side of true dark pink once it's buffed out. Pink One Piece, a neon, corally pink, is the lightest and most natural of the bunch when blended. Neon Pink is a bold, vivid, neon blue-based pink that gives major flush. Popo is a light purple lavender color and the hardest to pull off, but if you have a very light complexion it's cute and fresh. My Peach is exactly what it sounds like, a true peach color that's great for warming up pale skin.

3CE also has many, many, traditional powder color options—too many to name here—but I will tell you about some of my favorite shades I've tried. All That Peach is described as a "matte calm apricot" but it's my perfect warm peach shade. The blush is very finely milled and applies smoothly.

Love Filter is a pinky coral with pearlescent sheen, and it's what I wished NARS Orgasm looked like on me. It gives a beautiful, soft glow without being too orange or too pink.

Peach Sleeve is a soft apricot shade with a slight golden shimmer that's really good for the fairest of skins because it's almost impossible to overapply. It warms up your complexion without looking spray-tan-orange. The color is very soft, and while a blush that is not obviously pigmented is usually a detraction, in this case, it ends up working as a plus.

EYESHADOW

Since healthy skin and a smooth complexion are the main focus of Korean looks, the eyeshadows don't normally take a prominent role. When I first got into K-beauty, almost every shadow I tried was glittery, sparkly, and sheer. But that's not to say there aren't some wonderful formulations or vibrant, fun colors, because these certainly are.

The Face Shop Styling Triple Eyes

If you're looking for highly pigmented, finely milled, easily blendable shadows, The Face Shop Styling Triple Eyes are great little trios of eyeshadow that come in five selections. Brown Nuance, Orange Nuance, Grey Nuance, Violet Nuance, and Mocha Nuance. Mocha Nuance is a particular favorite of mine as it comes with two beautiful, warm, matte nudes, and one glittery gold highlight. It's the perfect blend of glamorous and low key, depending on which configuration you choose to wear them in. When I travel, I like to take this trio with me, since they go from day to night very easily.

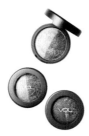

VDL Love Mark Festival Mineral Eyes

VDL is a brand that reminds me very much of MAC, both in packaging and in color choices. Their Festival Mineral Eyes (Love Mark) shadows are baked, shimmery, marbled shadows, that apply pigmented and smoothly with little fall-out. They are oversized, have two shades in a single pot, and lots of fun color choices. With names like N.Y. 34th Street, Sky Lounge, and Cafe Terrace, there are eight different duos to choose from, and none of them are boring. Made with a formula that catches the light, these are highly flattering, long-lasting, and a lot of fun.

Etude House Look At My Eyes

One of the things that never ceased to amaze me, is how Korean cosmetics, even the most budget-friendly of options, are of such high quality. Etude House, for example, has eye shadow singles that retail for $3.50, but perform just as well as eyeshadows I've paid $30 for. Etude House Look At My Eyes eyeshadow solo pots are highly pigmented, rich, velvety, and available in sixty different shades.

The Look At My Eyes collection is split into three different lines: Look At My Eyes, which comes in an array of finishes; Look At My Eyes Cafe, which contain eighteen beautiful matte selections, and Look At My Eyes Jewel, nineteen shades of sparkly pearl-finish shadows. No matter what you're looking for, there's bound to be something you'll love in this collection.

Etude House Eyeshadow Palettes

Etude House has been known to release limited edition palettes every year, sometimes every season, and they are always highly pigmented, on trend, and affordable. Some of my past limited-edition favorites (that are sadly no longer available) included Etude House & Rose Flowering Eyes, and Etude House Fantastic Color Eyes palettes. Be on the lookout for their palettes on their website, they always seem to be winners!

3 Concept Eyes Glam Cream Eyeshadows

If cream eyeshadows are your thing, 3CE Glam Cream Eyeshadows come in five different, long-lasting shades. You can apply these with a synthetic brush, or even your fingers for a more natural smudge.

The shade Golden Nude is one that I really like for light, quick eye looks. This shade would work on any skin tone, from the fairest to the darkest. Simply buff it onto your lid for a gorgeous slick of golden beige shimmer. Smoky Gray is a shade that can be used for a super-quick, but super-glam smoky eye. Pair it with a deep black liner and throw on a pair of false eyelashes and you're ready for a night out in no time. Golden Nude and Smoky Gray also pair quite well together, so if you have both, you can use them together to create a soft, fun look.

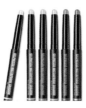

Clio Gelpresso Waterproof Pencil Shadows

If simplicity is your game, you'll love Clio Gelpresso Waterproof Pencil Shadows. I absolutely love these chubby pencils. They have proved their waterproof status to me in extreme conditions, and are exceedingly easy to blend and work with. Available in six shades with fun names like Beer Pong, Moving Lovings, Hold Me Tight, In Your Place, Bottoms Up, and In The Dark, they apply very pigmented and once they set, they stay.

For a pretty look reminiscent of the sky at sunset, use Hold Me Tight on the lid, blending the shadow into a gradient, then follow with Moving Love along the lower lids. It catches the light in the prettiest way and always gets compliments.

TonyMoly Crystal Stick Shadow

TonyMoly Crystal Stick Shadow has the same delivery system as the Clio Gelpresso Waterproof Pencil Shadows, but is a little different. Containing rosehip oil, vitamin C, vitamin A, and vitamin E, this stick shadow gives a softer wash of color. I especially like using shades #01 White Beam and #02 Luxury Gold, to highlight and create *aegyo sal* (more on that later in the makeup looks section!).

EYEBROW MAKEUP

Your eyebrows frame not only your eyes, but your entire face. A poorly shaped brow can make the most beautiful person look completely "off." A healthy, well-shaped, thicker brow takes center stage in Korean beauty.

This look dates all the way back to antiquity when aristocratic women of the Joseon era (1392–1897) would make a mixture of indigo plant ash, soot, and gold powder to enhance the eyebrow. Even the poorer commoners made it a point to give their brows the same attention the aristocrats did, substituting the expensive mixtures with cheap, easily found charcoal. There was even a handbook of sorts written in 1809 called 규합총서, *Gyuhap Chongseo*, or "Women's Encyclopedia," which gave all sorts of advice to women, including ten different fashionable shapes for eyebrows, the most popular being the "willow leaf" shapes.

The willow leaf is a long, thicker, straight shape, which has had a resurgence in popularity in Korea in recent years. The straight brow is all the rage right now, and the most desirable shape, as it's said to make one appear more youthful. Arched brows are not a very common naturally occurring shape amongst Koreans, so settling on this flatter, straight shape, makes sense. No matter what shape of eyebrow you choose, there are some amazing Korean products to help you get a beautiful brow, whether is be a pencil, powder, or "browcara," there are plenty of options to choose from.

The Face Shop Brow Master Eyebrow Kit

Starting with the traditional brow powders, I really like The Face Shop Brow Master Eyebrow Kit, a tiny little powder duo housed in a small, book-shaped compact. It also comes with an angle brush and spoolie, giving you everything you need to fill your brows. The powder is finely milled with nice pigmentation. It comes in two shades, 02 Beige Brown, a warm brown that would be suitable for blondes and lighter brunettes, and 01 Grey Brown, a cooler-toned darker brown. I like the Brow Master Eyebrow Kit because while they are pigmented, they're not too pigmented. Especially when attempting to fill in sparse brows, you don't want something too dark or you're going to look cartoonish. If you have naturally black brows, it's best to shade down a notch or two when trying to make brows bolder, but you want to avoid looking like Shin-Chan or Bert from Sesame Street.

Holika Holika Wonder Drawing Eyebrow Kit

Another great brow powder comes from the Holika Holika Wonder Drawing Eyebrow Kit. It's almost identical in formula and wear to The Face Shop version, but this kit is a trio, giving you three different colors in each compact. It also come with two brushes for application. Like The Face Shop's, this Holika Holika version is only available in two different shade choices, 01 Dark Brow and 02 Natural Brow.

Holika Holika Wonder Drawing 24hr Auto Eyebrow

Holika Holika has an entire line of different brow products in their Wonder line. There's also a great little brow pencil line called Wonder Drawing 24hr Auto Eyebrow. This pencil comes in a larger range of shades including 01 Grey Black, 02 Dark Brown, 03 Light Brown, and 04 Red Brown.

The Auto Eyebrow is an automatic twist-up type pencil with a unique, flat, slanted edge. It makes drawing in your eyebrows so much easier compared to a traditional pencil point. It also features a spoolie at the other end of the pencil so that you can comb and blend the color into your brows. The 03 Light Brown shade in this line would work really well for blondes and light brunettes, while 02 Dark Brown works well for darker brunettes.

Holika Holika Wonder Drawing 1 Sec Finish Browcara

Also in the line is the Holika Holika Wonder Drawing 1 Sec Finish Browcara. What is a browcara? It's exactly what it sounds like, a mascara-type product for the brows. A browcara both grooms and colors brows as you brush it on, and this formula promises to dry quickly without smudging. The packaging looks like a small mascara wand, with a brush head about a quarter of the length of a mascara. This browcara is highly pigmented and available in three shades, #1 Natural Brown, #2 Light Brown, #3 Red Brown, and #4 Dark Brown.

It's possible to go overboard with a browcara, so please apply lightly at first until you're comfortable with the way it goes on and the opacity.

There are several Korean brands with their own browcara formulations, so if one brand doesn't work for you, don't give up just yet, there are plenty more to try. Etude House, The Saem, Banila Co, PeriPera, Nature Republic, and Innisfree all have their own versions. Eyebrows are serious business in Korea!

Etude House Tint My Brow

Another brow product formula available is the brow tint. Etude House Tint My Brow is one of the more budget-friendly ways to try out a brow tint; it retails at well under $10 USD and is available in two shades, #1 Gray Brown and #2 Natural Brown.

Brow tints usually stain the skin (like a lip tint or stain) and offer a natural tint to fill in the brow. They're long lasting, but not very dramatic. Some people like to start with a base of a brow tint for definition, and then follow up with a pencil or browcara to change the overall color of the brows. Brow tints usually have a fine point tip like a liquid eyeliner pen to deliver a precise application. Some tints claim to last for twenty-four hours; some claim to last for days.

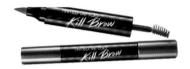

Clio Tinted Tattoo Kill Brow

Another option is the Clio Tinted Tattoo Kill Brow, which manages to combine both the tint and the browcara into one handy tube. The tint end has a fine-tipped, but chubbier nib compared to the Etude House Tint. On the other end it has a matching shade of browcara.

Clio Tinted Tattoo Kill Brow claims to last for up to two days, even after washing your face. While that's partially true, I find that a good oil cleanser will remove the tint. Still, it is very long lasting and good to wear if you're going swimming or doing intense activity.

This product is available in three shades: #1 Earth Brown, a soft light neutral brown; #2 Soft Brown, which has more of a red tint, and #3 Dark Brown, which is a dark, ashy brown. I especially like that it is a combination product, so it's travel-friendly. Whenever I go on long trips this always makes its way into my makeup bag.

EYELINER

Korean eyeliners are, in short, amazing. When I'm trying to get someone to convert to K-beauty, eyeliners are always my gateway product. Once someone tries my liner recommendations, they inevitably come to me saying, "OMG, show me more!"

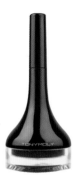

TonyMoly Backstage Gel Eyeliner

For instance, I used to swear by Mac's Fluidline. I would buy two at a time just to ensure I would never be without it. That all changed one day when I ended up running out unexpectedly due to an unscrewed cap dying out the product. In a panic, I went to the Korean cosmetics store located across the street from my building in a search of a gel eyeliner. I came across a very interesting glass pot with a detachable brush built into the lid that looked like a minimalistic genie bottle. Upon further inspection I saw that this product looked exactly like my beloved Fluidline, so I quickly purchased it and ran back across the street to finish my makeup.

Wow. The formulation is buttery, smooth, applies without dragging, and was an even deeper, richer black that my former gel liner. As if that wasn't enough, it was even more tenacious than the Fluidline.

Let me give you an example: I am a practitioner of hot yoga. That means I do sixty- to ninety-minute long classes in temperatures of 105°F (40.6°C). I often head into class at night wearing the makeup I applied that morning. When I exit class, after copious amounts of sweating and exertion, my eyeliner remains as flawless as when I first applied it. It does not budge. It doesn't even come off in the shower unless I first remove it with a balm or oil-type cleanser. This product is amazing.

It's available in your typical shade range, from black, to brown, to grey, with seasonal colors sometimes released in limited edition. I'm also a fan of the built-in brush: it's flat, slightly wider than a fine-point liner brush, and it works especially well for doing a puppy-dog eyeliner look. If there was just a single product I would recommend to you in this book, it would be the TonyMoly Backstage Gel Eyeliner. Seriously, it's a must try.

Clio Waterproof Kill Liner

If you prefer liquid liner to gel, Clio Waterproof Kill Liner is what you're looking for. This fine-tipped liquid pen liner is tenacious: no running, no flaking, and once it's set, no smearing. It's available in two shades, Kill Black and Kill Brown, and both are very deep, rich colors. Lots of people are singing its praises for staying put and never creating the dreaded raccoon eye.

Etude House Play 101 Pencil

Coming in at a close second for my favorite eyeliner product is the Etude House Play 101 Pencil. These wonderful little multifunctional pencils come in fifty shades with five different finishes (creamy, matte, glossy, shimmering, and glitter). The different finishes have different properties and recommended uses.

From the Etude House website, "Creamy" is described as "soft drawing texture with rich colors," shades #1 and #50, which are a rich black and darkest brown, and are my picks for that finish.

"Matte" is "soft drawing but powdery finish." Recommended for use as eyebrow, eyeshadow, concealer, and base, #08 is a perfect, heavy concealer for me that I use in the inner corners of my eyes next to my nose. I also like shade #42 as a brow pencil. Shimmering and glitter finishes are exactly what they sound like. The shimmery and glittery colors include some of the best highlighter shades I've ever used: #6 and #28 are notable choices.

The finish "Glossy" is "recommended for use as blusher or lips." I love making my own lipsticks with all of their glossy shades. I customize them by making them lighter or darker with the #08 or #50 shade to create the color I want.

When I say they're multipurpose, they're truly multipurpose. You could do a whole look with just pencils. In fact, the famous Korean YouTube personality, and makeup artist, Pony, has several tutorials online showing exactly how to do that. They're worth a Google for some great inspiration.

Another neat thing about this liner is that it has a removable sharpener built into the back of the pencil. It's like a little self-contained makeup kit, with everything you need on the go.

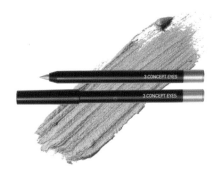

3 Concept Eyes Under Eye Flash

In many popular Korean eye looks, dark lower liner is passed over in favor of a bright flash of liner, usually in a neutral tone. This is to make the eye appear bigger, brighter, and more lively. Just as a dark liner makes light eyes pop, bright, highlighter-type liner makes dark eyes flash with brilliance. But your eyes needn't be dark to make this look work. It also makes for a sweet, innocent, wide-eyed look, which is good for days that you need to look alert, no matter what your eye color is.

3 Concept Eyes Under Eye Flash does exactly that. Long-lasting and waterproof, this "flash" liner glides on smooth and lasts all day long. I love this line and ended up purchasing all six available shades.

My favorite is #1 Romanticism, a brilliant pinky beige. It makes for a gorgeous, coppery neutral look that's anything but boring. #4 Brown Sugar, a creamy beige, is another beautiful shade that's great for test-driving the fresh, sans-dark-lower-liner-look. #06 African Sunset, a burgundy rust color, is a bit more dramatic. Applied on the top and bottom lid, and then smudged, it gives you a new twist on smoky.

Clio Gelpresso Waterproof Pencil Gel Liner

Another Clio product I'd be remiss not to mention is Clio Gelpresso Waterproof Pencil Gel Liner. This is the sister product of the Clio Gelpresso Waterproof Pencil Shadow we touched on earlier. This gel liner is in pencil form, and like the TonyMoly Gel Liner, has serious waterproof lasting power.

These Gelpresso Eyeliners don't have any traditional eyeliner colors so speak. For example, you won't find a matte black or brown shade. There is, however, a black flecked with gold glitter, and a glittery brown. The other colors are a shimmery beige, jade, and silver, along with a glittery khaki, purple, and navy.

This automatic twist-up pencil also has a built in detachable sharpener like the Etude House Play 101 Pencils. They certainly don't have the range of shades that the Play 101 Pencils do, and they aren't as multipurpose, but they smoothly apply very saturated colors, and shine brilliantly when they catch the light. I love using the shimmery shades to highlight the inner corners of my eyes.

Etude House Tear Drop Liner

When I'm looking for the most dramatic eye highlight possible, I like to turn to the liquid glitter liner products that have been the hallmark for Korean eye looks for some years with young women. Etude House Tear Drop Liner is a liquid liner packed with micro glitter meant to be applied outside around the tear duct area in the inner corner of your eyes.

Unlike the pure shimmer highlights that come in pencil form, this liquid liner has a more intense glitter effect. Definitely not for a wallflower, these are fun and the sparkle is attention grabbing. These are also nice to pair with smoky eye looks for that added oomph and drama when going out at night. The crystalized look also pairs well with a neutral eye for a sweet, pretty, innocent look.

You're not just limited to a pure white with these: there are four dazzling shades available, a crystal white, a pink pearl type, an opal, and even a light golden bronze.

MASCARA

The finishing touch to any eye look is probably the most important: mascara. Nobody looks finished without mascara. It's probably the product you'd choose to wear should you be limited to only one.

I struggled for a long time to find a Korean mascara that really spoke to me. It was the last Korean product that I made the switch to. I was very partial to the gigantic, fluffy brushes common to European and North American mascara companies. I had it in my head that I couldn't get the volume I wanted without them, and I was paying close to $40 a tube without batting a lash (ha).

As soon as I found my favorite Korean mascaras, I was mad at all the money I'd wasted over the years on the expensive stuff. Not that there's anything wrong with treating yourself to a little luxury, but I was spending that much thinking I had to in order to get the results I wanted. The Korean mascaras I found gave me everything I wanted, at a fraction of the cost. As was proven to me, time and time again, the Korean versions were just as good, if not better than what I previously used.

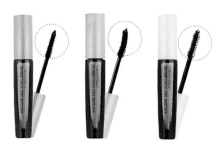

TonyMoly Circle Lens Mascara

The first Korean mascara that I recommend to people is also the best deal out there. TonyMoly Circle Lens Mascara retails at just under $5, and performs just as well as my $30+ tubes. The Circle Lens Mascara line is named as such because it's meant to make your eyes look defined and dramatic, like when you're wearing eye-enhancing circle contact lenses.

It comes in three versions: #1 Volume Circle, #2 Curling & Long Lash Circle, and #3 Clear Circle. Volume Circle creates serious volume with a precision, bullet-shaped brush, and is my favorite version since I'm a volume junkie. #2 Curling & Long Lash Circle has a curved banana-shaped brush that builds nice length and curl. #3 Clear Circle is a clear mascara meant to be used as sealant, or you could use it as I do, on the brows after filling them in with powder or pencil. If you'd like to define your lower lashes but always manage to get mascara all over and under your eyes, the clear version is a good way to do that mess-free.

Although these are not waterproof, they do stay put and don't flake or smear easily. And yet, they remove pretty easily, which is good news to those of you concerned about irritation or unnecessary roughness around the delicate eye skin during removal.

It's Skin Babyface Mascara

Another great mascara option is from the brand It's Skin. It's Skin Babyface Mascara comes in a cute little tube with a cartoon winky face, and brags that its formula contains aloe, soy, royal jelly, and gives moisture and nutrition to lashes. Available in two different options—Volume Setting and Long & Curling—and both do exactly what they claim. The finish is natural and not overly dramatic, but not at all wimpy. This mascara also has the added benefit of being a great choice for those with sensitive eyes.

The Face Shop Face It All About Mascara

Rounding out my favorites is The Face Shop Face It All About Mascara line. It comes in six different types, Transparent, Power Volume, Power Curl, Long Long, Mini Power, and Under Lash, which comes with a mini brush for lower lashes.

My two picks from this line are definitely Mini Power, which is great for people with small straight lashes since it has a thin brush that easily grips puny lashes, and Long Long, which is a fiber mascara that makes for some serious length. Out of the six different options, there's bound to be one that works for you.

LIP COLOR

Whether it be a natural flush or something a little more daring, Korean lip products are one of my very favorite things to shop for. You can change your whole mood with a good lipstick. Ranging from the extremely cute (TonyMoly Petite Bunny Gloss Bars) to modern and sophisticated (VDL Expert Color Lip Cube), Korean brands offer just about anything you could ever ask for in a lip color.

Korean lip products aren't just limited to run-of-the-mill lipsticks or glosses, there are many unique formulas that are currently enjoying a lot of popularity. Thanks to the gradient lip trend, stains are particularly sought after to achieve this look. Since the original gradient lip was meant to look as though you have just eaten a popsicle, a stain works particularly well to mimic that effect.

Applied only on the innermost part of the top and bottom lip, and then either left alone or gone over with a lighter gloss, this is the default gradient look. You can also apply all over for a sexy dark color wash that won't smudge.

The Face Shop's Lovely Me: Ex My Lips Eat Cherry Aqua Tint

I particularly enjoy The Face Shop's Lovely Me: Ex My Lips Eat Cherry Aqua Tint. It has a watery consistency that stains lips perfectly without drying them out. There is little to no transfer of this product onto cups or straws, so it's great to wear while out to a coffee or a lunch date.

There are three shades, 01 Juicy Cherry, which honestly reads as tomato orange, 02 Juicy Red, which when blended looks like a darker hot pink but can build to a pinky red; and 03 Bloody Red, which is a deeper, more burgundy tint.

While they don't explicitly say so, you can use these tints as blushes as well. I've used these on set when I want a naturally flushed look.

The Face Shop Lovely Me: Ex The Aqua Proof Marker Tint

Also from The Face Shop Lovely Me: Ex lineup is the Aqua Proof Marker Tint. I love this tint for two reasons, the cute natural stain it gives, and the unique applicator. It's housed in what looks exactly like a magic marker, and I suppose it is, of sorts, only it goes on your lips instead of on paper.

This tint is water-based so it's not sticky or tacky, it doesn't smudge or smear at all once it sets, and it sets pretty much instantly. My personal recommendation would be the shade 02 Pink, which is a really flattering, true baby pink. It's hard to get that shade right, and this one is cute without being childish. There's only one other shade available in this tint and that's 01 Cherry, which is also a very nice choice.

This tint marker lasts and lasts; however, it can dry out your lips a bit, so I would recommend you apply a balm beforehand. The finish is matte, but if you're into shine, popping a gloss on over this looks great.

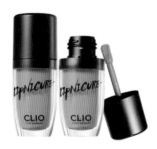

Clio Virgin Kiss Lipnicure

If you want all of the staying power of a tint, but with the intense color of a lipstick, you absolutely must try the Clio Virgin Kiss Lipnicure. If you're wondering what a "Lipnicure" is, you're not alone. When I first heard about this product I had to look it up myself. Apparently it's a marriage of the words manicure and lipstick, as this product claims it has the staying power of a manicure.

Let me go ahead and confirm that for you: it really does. Once this liquid lipstick is applied to your lips and sets, it ain't goin' nowhere. Completely transfer-proof, waterproof, and smudge proof, this is one hell of a tenacious lippie. You have to use an oil-based remover to fully erase all traces of it.

I would recommend the darker hues in the thirteen-shade line, as I find the lightest shades tend to apply patchy. #8 Guilty Pink is probably my favorite; I like to wear this when I'm going on dinner dates, as it's a fun, bold color, and unless I'm eating something greasy like fried chicken, isn't going to budge.

Lipnicure applies with slight shine at first, but dries to a matte finish. It doesn't necessarily dry out your lips, but make sure you apply balm beforehand.

There is also another version of the Lipnicure that offers a high-gloss finish. Clio Lipnicure Glass gives you all of the staying power of the original matte Lipnicure, all of the gloss of a lipgloss, and none of the stickiness.

3 Concept Eyes Creamy Lip Color

Speaking of gloss, there's a lip product I love by 3 Concept Eyes that straddles the line between gloss and lipstick perfectly. Traditional tube glosses have fallen out of fashion as of late, but if you still want all the moisture and shine without any of the sticky feel, then I encourage you to give 3 Concept Eyes Creamy Lip Color a try.

Whereas the lip glosses of yore were tacky to the touch, the Creamy Lip Color glides on like melting butter, leaving behind a glossy shine. It comes in a slim lipstick form, and boasts a formula that is made up of twenty percent moisturizing ingredients such as argan oil and cupuacu butter, so your lips are left incredibly soft and supple. Don't expect a lot of staying power from a formula this rich and creamy, but it does impart a vivid flash of color.

I absolutely love this product and own almost every shade, of which there are twelve to choose from. Notable favorites are #2 Cotton Pie, which is a wonderful warm nude, and #9 Kitsch Biker, a dazzling, insanely bright, head-turning, orange-based red.

3 Concept Eyes Lip Lacquer
3 Concept Eyes also makes another favorite of mine that occupies several worlds at once. 3 Concept Eyes Lip Lacquer is a liquid-type product, housed in a tube (like a gloss), has the thick consistency of a lacquer, and gives intense color like a lipstick. It's applied with a doe-foot wand and dries to a semi-matte, powdery finish with a slight kick of shine. It's not forgiving to dry lips like the Creamy Lip Color (so be sure your lips are exfoliated and moisturized before application), but it does have more lasting power.

My favorite shade out of the 10 available is Bon Bon. It's one of the most fun nude type hues I can think of, falling somewhere between a pinky brown and a salmon color, and it gives lips an unexpected twist on neutral.

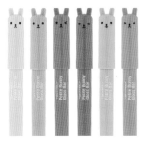

TonyMoly Petite Bunny Gloss Bar
If something cute and light is what you're looking for, you can't get any cuter than TonyMoly Petite Bunny Gloss Bar. Even its scent is sweet and cute! It comes in a slim tube and each lid has is shaped like a little bunny head, each with a different facial expression. It applies semi-sheer like a gloss, and comes in nine adorable shades.

Pulling this gloss bar out of your makeup bag, you're guaranteed to elicit grins from everyone around you. It's impossible to swipe this across your lips and be in a bad mood. I love giving these out as gifts, they're both functional and smile inducing. How many products can you say that about?

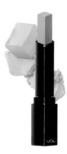

VDL Expert Color Lip Cube SPF 10

I'd like to close out this section out by introducing you to my favorite lipstick—not just my favorite Korean lipstick—but my favorite lipstick period. VDL Expert Color Lip Cube SPF 10 is hands-down my holy grail lipstick. I think the VDL Cosmetics website says it best: "The architectural depth of color and shape created by the lines and planes of the cube takes the lipstick to a whole new level. Enhanced with a luxurious, velvety texture and long-lasting, elegant colors defined with cubic edges, VDL Expert Color Lip Cube presents to you inimitable attitude and confidence".

The gimmick of the square-cubed lipstick bullet drew me in, but the sophisticated, luxurious, color palette and formulation kept me coming back time and time again. The packaging is very sturdy and sleek; you can tell it's not cheaply made, especially in comparison to lower-end offerings. The lipstick itself applies like a dream and has a very high-end, luxury-brand feel. It has a faint sweet floral scent that I find so pleasant.

The color selection is so gorgeous, there's not a dud in the bunch; they're all winners. The jewel-toned shades coat your lips in a rich color, and the lighter shades are never, ever boring. Shade 101 Witch Flower is my power lipstick. When I attend important meetings or need to feel like a boss, this is my go-to shade. It's both sexy and powerful: I love it! I'm also a big fan of the deep, rich red found in shade 501 Outbloom.

Not only is the unexpected lipstick shape cool to look at, but the cube's edges make applying this lipstick very easy and precise around tricky areas like the cupid's bow.

You would think that with such a pigmented intense color, these lipsticks might dry the lips. Not so. They are actually very plush and cushy. There is just so much to love here!

This lipstick does cost a bit more than a lot of other Korean lipsticks, retailing at around $20, but it's worth its price. I've never once pulled this out of my bag and not had someone who's not familiar with it make eyes at it and ask me questions. I absolutely adore this lipstick and can't speak highly enough of it—it's an absolute must try.

So, that was our walk through the alluring world of Korean makeup. After introducing you to some of my favorites, I hope you're inspired you to get out there and discover your own treasures. The beautiful frustration of the innovation of the Korean beauty world is that by the time this book goes to press, I'll know I'll have discovered a hundred new products I'd wish I could share with you.

Now, let's take a peek at some beautiful Korean-style inspired makeup looks I've put together for you!

SEMI-MATTE LOOK

Fear not, those of you who lived through the 90s. This is not that heavily powdered, absorbing all light and goodness around you, flat-matte look that had a resurgence lasting into the early 2000s. This matte look is much sweeter, and has a real softness to it, thanks to strategic highlighting. Really it's the best of both worlds, thanks to Korea's popular take on it. There is a really warm sultriness to this look that reminds me of old, golden-age Hollywood.

Apply a matte finish BB cream or foundation, then softly highlight around the C-zones of the orbital bone, across the forehead, and down the nose bridge. A powder highlight would work best here, but a cream or liquid applied with a light hand will work in a pinch.

Here our model is wearing:
- Missha M Perfect Cover BB cream in #27 mixed with a tiny bit of #31.
- To really showcase her flawless matte skin, there is no blush, only highlight, which was done with a very light hand (fingers actually), using the Innisfree Mineral Glow Stick (such a handy product!).
- The eyeshadow is The Face Shop Face It Styling Triple Eyes in Mocha Nuance, topped off by TonyMoly Backstage Gel Eyeliner in black, and The Face Shop Face It All About Mascara in Long Lash on the top lashes only.
- The lower lids are swiped with the golden highlight shade from the Mocha Nuance trio, and bottom mascara was skipped for a softer look.
- Her lips, which imake this look so glamourous, were done with VDL Festival Lipstick (Love Mark) in Matte Intense 502 Cruz.

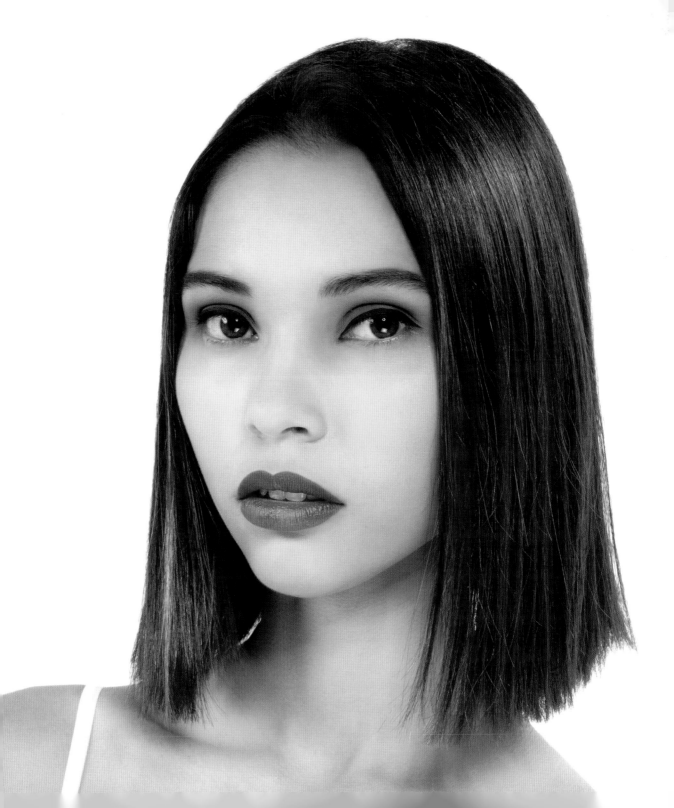

This look is perfect for your next date night. It's alluring, sexy, and it absolutely smolders.

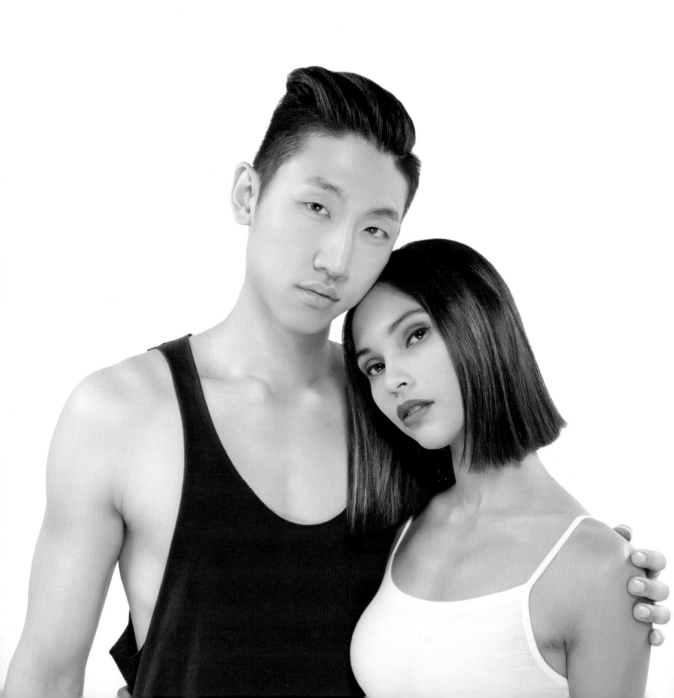

SUNRISE/SUNSET

These two looks are variations of what we see at the two most beautiful times of day, sunrise and sunset. The brilliant oranges that emerge as the sun rises into the sky, signifying a fresh new start for us all. Later, as our day comes to a close, it's almost as if the sky is celebrating all that we've accomplished, and rewards us with a light show of beautiful pinks, both dusky and bright.

I've seen a lot of pink and orange looks and makeup collections from Korea. They're so beautiful and can work on anyone. In fact, I saw looks very similar to these on a Korean beauty show. The minute I saw them I knew they could work on a much wider range of skin tones than they were demonstrated on, and I think they translated wonderfully.

Our model, Laureen, on the left is our pink sunset princess, and she's wearing:

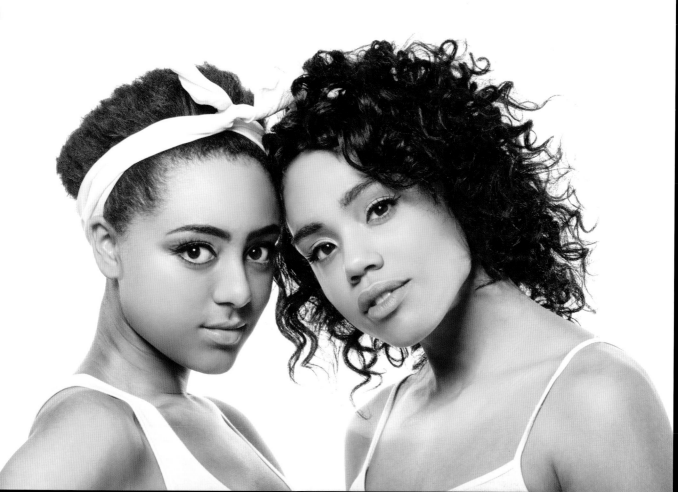

- Missha M Cover foundation in #27 with a drop of #31 and the most important, key product to create this look, the Etude House House Precious Mineral Magic Any Cushion primer in the shade Pink. I took this primer and applied a generous layer using not the silicon puff it came with, but a flat foundation brush. I blended it into the cheeks and across the bridge of the nose, creating a soft pink wash of color.
- From there, I used The Face Shop My Lips Eat Cherry Aqua Tint both as blush and on the lips, applied with my fingers.
- The eyeshadow is from the Etude House Fantastic Color Eyes Cherry Blossom palette, and the liner is TonyMoly Backstage Gel Eyeliner in Black.

Amelie on the right is channeling the cheerful warm sunrise with her orange look. She's wearing:

- Missha M Cover foundation in #31.
- We used The Face Shop Lovely ME:EX Pastel Cushion Blusher in Coral for the blush.
- For the eyes we paired Clio Pro Single Shadow in shades Peony, Teeny Tiny, and Brazilian with Clio Waterproof Pen Liner in Kill Black.
- We then did a gradient on her gorgeous, full lips using Peripera Peri's Tint Crayon in 05 Fruity Sunny.

Two gorgeous looks plucked right from the sky!

We loved the orange look so much we wanted to show you a variation of it on our model Lanny. Here we demonstrate how universally flattering orange can be. Lanny is wearing:

- Skin prepped with The Face Shop Mango Seed Glow Date-Prep Cream, followed by Peripera Watery Face Pride Up Cushion Pact in 01 Peach Beige
- We then highlighted her face with Etude House Nymph Aura Volumer for an ultra dewy look.
- Her brows were shaped with Clio Tinted Tattoo Kill Brow in Soft Brown
- Etude House Proof 10 Eye Primer was used on the lid, then L'Ocean Eyeshadow

in Pastel Orange was patted directly onto the eyes with Clio Waterproof Pen Liner in Kill Black along the upper lashline. The bottom lids were lined with Clio Gelpresso Waterproof Pencil Gel Liner in 01 Beige Shine.

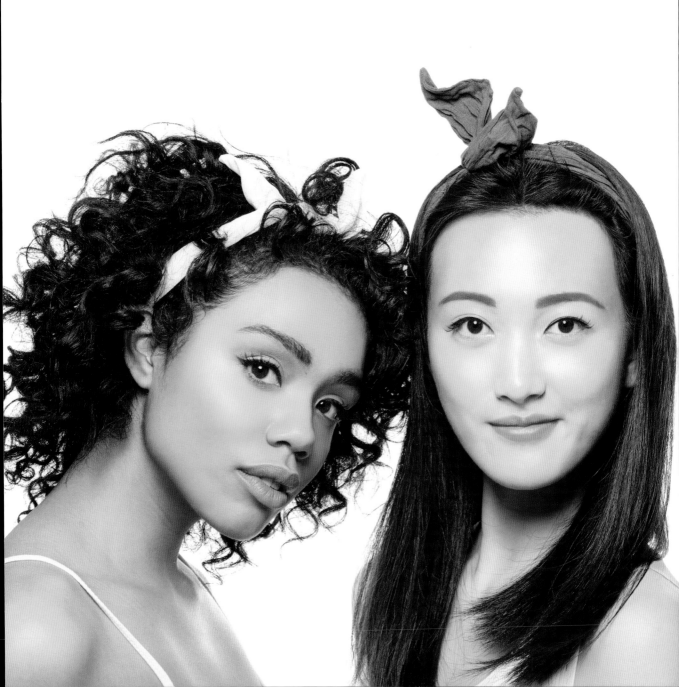

GWAPYEON (FRUITS CAKE)

This look reminds me of *Gwapyeon*, the little jellylike cakes made of fruit served on special occasions. However, you certainly don't need a special occasion to break out this simple look. Here Lea is showing how sweet simple can be!

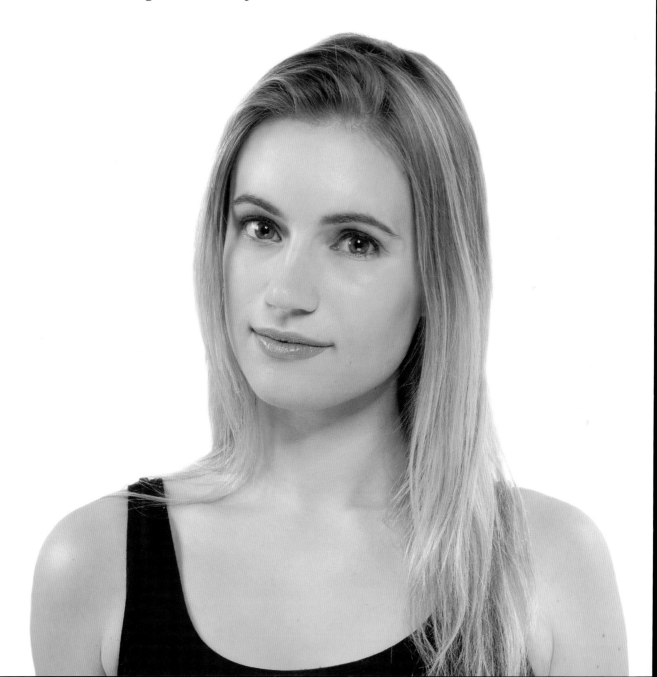

- To give our model Lea this sweet look, we started off by prepping her skin with a fine mist of Whamisa's Organic Flowers Olive Leaf Mist, then applying Missha's M Magic Cushion in #21.
- Her eyebrows were filled with The Face Shop Brow Master Eyebrow Kit in Beige Brown.
- We then took 3 Concept Eyes Under Eye Flash and lined her upper and lower eyelids, putting extra emphasis on the lower lid.
- We then laid down a very thin line of brown eyeliner with TonyMoly Backstage Gel Liner.
- Her cheeks were patted with The Face Shop Lovely Me: Ex Pastel Cushion Blusher in Peach Cushion and a little bit of highlight was given with the Nature Republic Botanical Stick Highlighter in 02.
- Tying everything together is 3 Concept Eyes Creamy Lip Color in Cotton Pie.

WATERCOLOR ROSE

This look is as delicate and pretty as a rose petal. The secret to keeping things as soft as a watercolor painting is keeping every finish matte, skipping the use of eyeliner, and forgoing any highlighters.

- Here Hue Linh lets her perfect skin speak volumes with the soft matte finish of the Missha M Magic Cushion in #23, and we took the matte finish one step further by applying a light dusting of Innisfree No Sebum Mineral Powder.
- Hue Linh's eyebrows were then filled and color softened with Holika Holika Wonder Drawing Eyebrow Kit in Natural Brow.
- We brushed TonyMoly Crystal Blusher in Pink Jubilee on the cheeks.
- Our makeup artist Chloe then buffed on TonyMoly Delight Mono Shadow Matte in #11 Vintage Coral, taking it all over and under her eyelid, making a very soft smoke.
- To give a bit of definition to the lashline without actually applying liner to the lid, Chloe tightlined the upper eyelashes with Etude House Play 101 Pencil in #50.
- It's Skin Babyface Mascara in Long & Curling Black was applied to the upper but not lower lashes, again to maintain a watercolor softness.
- Her lips were patted with 3 Concept Eyes Lip Crayon in Blushed, and violà, an edgy but soft look fit for a queen.

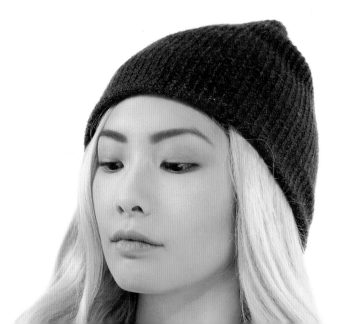

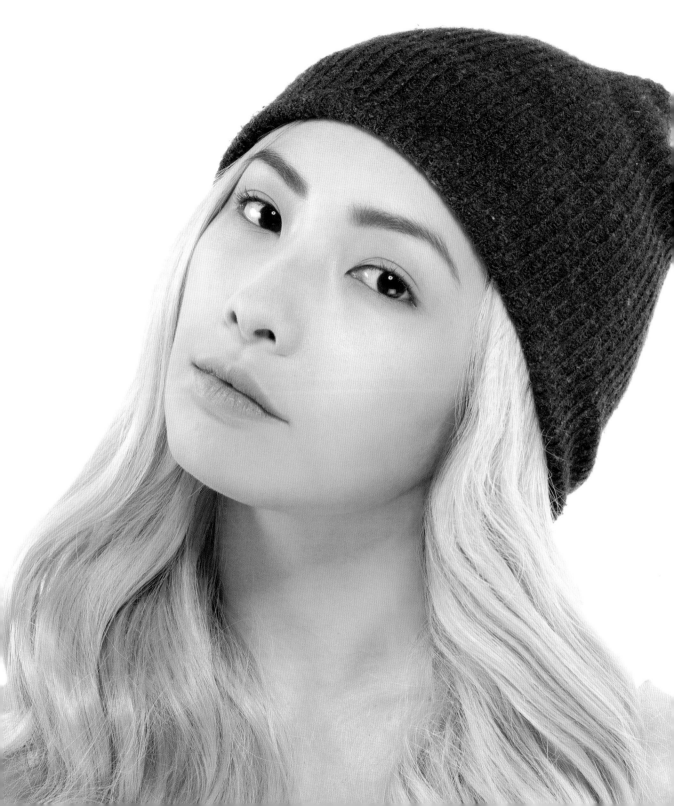

NIGHT ROSE

You can also build on this look and take it from day to night with a few additions.

- Here we started with the Watercolor Rose look, added some false eyelashes, and lined the upper and lower lashes with TonyMoly Backstage Gel Liner in Black.
- We also gave a bit of highlight with the Innisfree Mineral Glow Stick around the C-zones, nose, and cupid's bow.
- A shimmering highlight under the eyes was provided by a slick of TonyMoly Crystal Stick Eyeshadow in Champagne Pink.
- We gave a gradient lip with Clio Tension Lip in Pinkyely applied in the center of her lips, and then the outer edges of her lips were given a light coat of 3 Concept Eyes Creamy Lip Color in Rollercoaster.

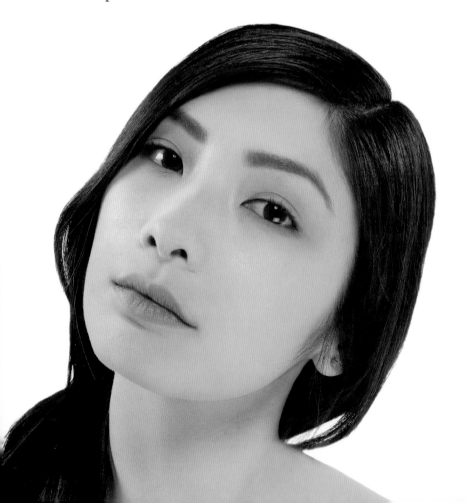

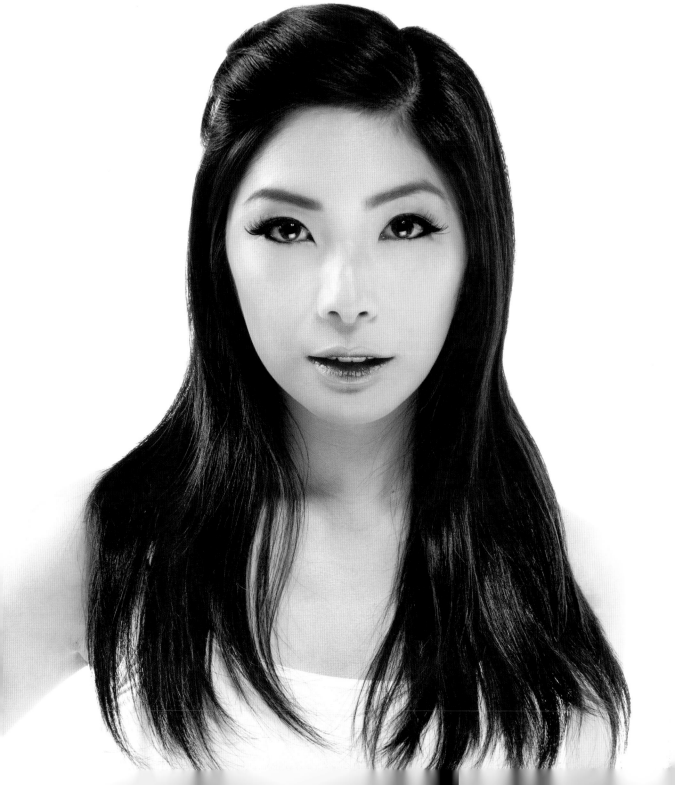

AEGYO SAL

There's been a huge trend in Korea for quite some time that involves eye bags. No, not the dark unwanted visitors we get when we neglect our sleep, but instead the cute bags of fat underneath the eyes that you often see in babies and young children. These little pockets of fat are called *aegyo sal* in Korean, which roughly translates to "baby eye fat." You see, almost everyone starts off life with aegyo sal, but some people lose it with age; therefore it's believed that still retaining the under-eye fat makes one more cute and youthful in appearance. There's even a popular plastic surgery in Korea to restore or create agyo sal!

Thankfully, you don't have to do something that dramatic to give yourself your own cute little baby eyes. Here we took Hue Linh after her Night Rose look and showed her how to fake the aygeo sal look with a cream-contouring product and highlighter. It's crazy simple!

- As you could see in her Night Rose look, Hue Linh doesn't have agyeo sal naturally, so we mimicked the raised look of the fat with the same TonyMoly Crystal Stick Eyeshadow in Champagne Pink we used before, just applied thicker and slightly heavier.
- We then took the Yeondukong x Memebox Easy Shading Stick in 01 Brown (a wonderful product) and applied it with a pointed liner brush, and viola! A super cute, and super easy Korean trend!

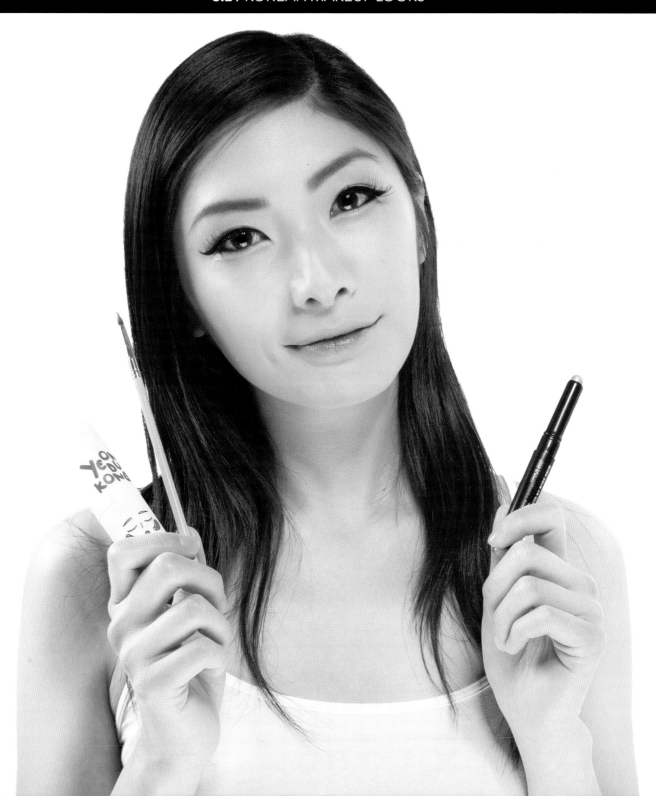

GRADIENT LIP & BLUSH

We talked about the gradient lip look in the lipstick section, well, there's also the next level, gradient blush! This look is very fashion forward, but anyone can pull it off! Here Sarah shows us how cute a full gradient look can be.

- We started off with a neutral eye look, so that the blush and lip could take center stage. For that we used The Face Shop Face It Styling Triple Eyes in Brown Nuance and then gave a bit of highlight under the eyes by lining them with Clio's Gelpresso Waterproof Pencil Gel Liner in Beige Shine.
- Then the fun part: we applied a two different The Face Shop Lovely Me: Ex Pastel Cushion Blusher blush colors, on the top in Rose, and on the bottom, Coral. The trick to this look is blending the two colors into each other, so you don't have a severe 80s-style blush stripe.
- For the gradient lip we applied The Face Shop Enamel Coating Tint in 01 Red Enamel (which I absolutely love the finish of). We applied it only on the innermost part of the lip, blending slightly with our fingers, and left the rest of the lip clean.

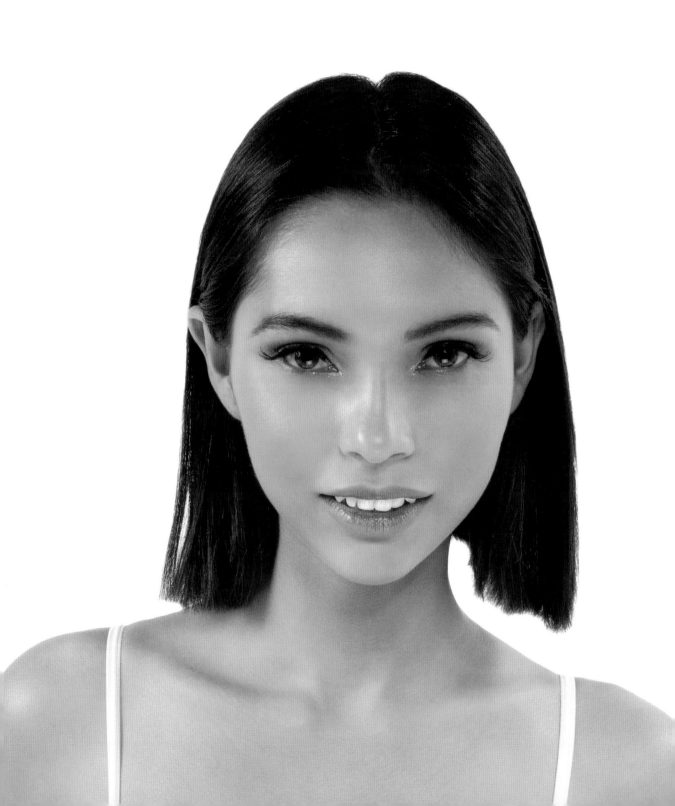

We also have Hue Linh showing off a slightly softer take on the gradient lip & gradient blush duo.

- She's wearing a single, softly applied eyeshadow, TonyMoly Eyetone Matte in shade M04.
- She has a soft cat eye applied with Clio Waterproof Pen Liner Kill Black and her lashes are coated with It's Skin Babyface Mascara 02 Volume Setting Black.
- Her lower lids are kept soft, lined with Clio Gelpresso Waterproof Pencil Shadow in #1 Make Me Up. For the gradient blush we used TonyMoly Cristal Blusher in #10 Orange and #11 Hot Pink.
- For that perfect, soft, effortless gradient lip we had a little trick up our sleeves: the Laneige Two Tone Lip Bar, an ingenious glossy lipstick that comes with two complimentary shades in a single bar. It makes a foolproof, perfect gradient every single time. There are ten shades available; here we used a beautiful orange paired with a light salmon pink that echoes the gradient blush perfectly, shade #3 Pink Salmon.

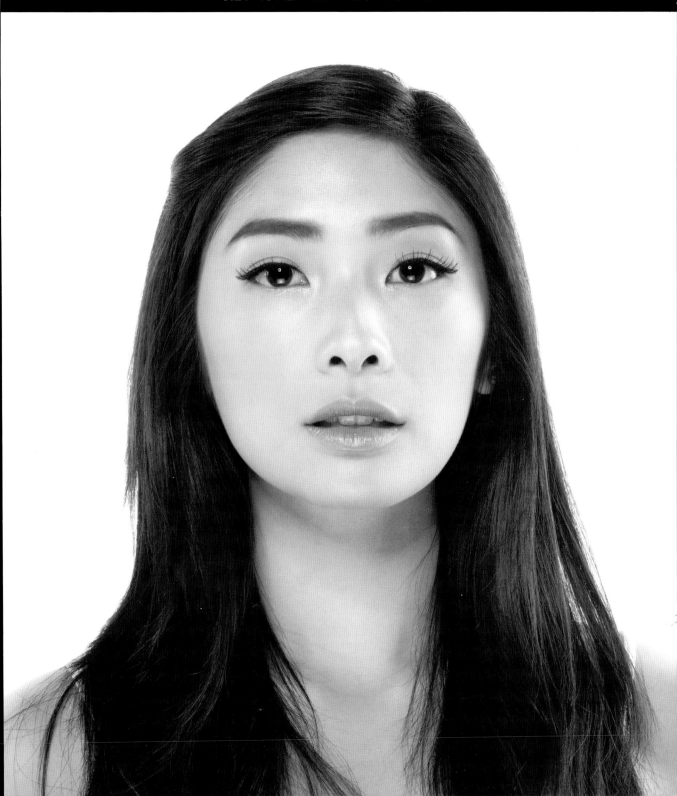

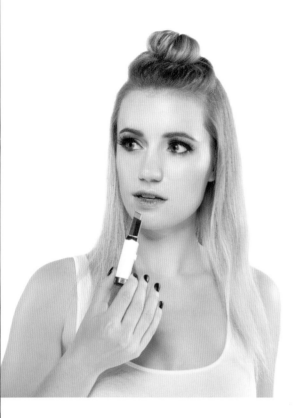

Here we have Lea showing the Laneige Two Tone Lip Bar in shade #10 Burgundy Love. Perfect gradient, perfect color, just perfect, period.

Getting back to Sarah's original gradient look, we can take it to the next level. By simply filling in the lips with a vivid color, it can take this fun look into something a little more sexy. A small tweak can completely change this look into something less casual, making it perfect for a daytime date or anytime you want some seductive sizzle.

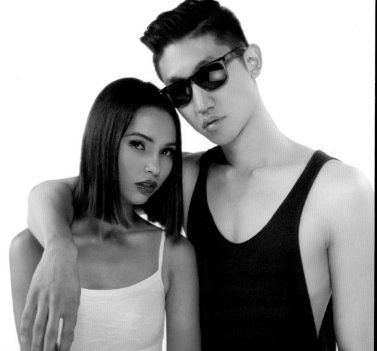

Here Sarah is kicking this look into high gear by applying The Face Shop Real Gloss Vivid Vibrant in Red Hommage all over the lip.

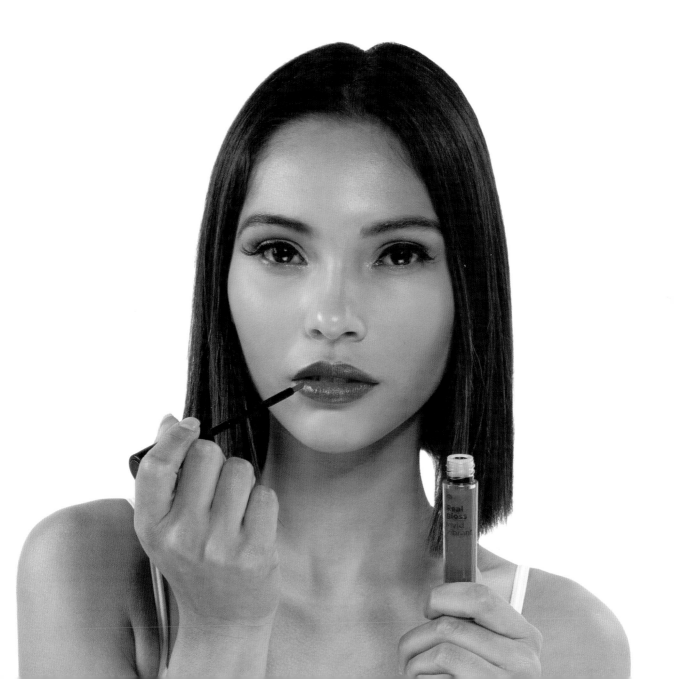

BAD GIRL

While I have you in the seductive mindset, let's take a look at an expression of seductive with serious edge. The Bad Girl look is inspired by a K-pop video whose visuals grabbed my eye immediately the first time I saw it. The look was edgy, sexy, raw, and fierce, which is everything I love.

- To get this look we prepped Hana's gorgeous skin with The Face Shop Mango Seed Glow Date-Prep Cream.
- We then used Missha's M Magic Cushion in #21 on her face, followed by Nymph Aura Volumer for a sexy glow.
- We added flush to her cheeks with Three Concept Eyes Face Blush in My Muse.
- Her eyebrows were defined with the Holika Holika Wonder Drawing 24hr Auto Eyebrow in 02 Dark Brown.
- We then smoked her eyes with VDL Festival Mineral Eyes (Love Mark) in 201 Central Park, and the Pony x Memebox Shine Easy Glam palette.
- Her eyelids were given a thick, sloping line of TonyMoly Backstage Gel Liner in Black.
- We then went for maximum drama by attaching two pairs of false eyelashes to her lids, making sure to curl both pairs together with an eyelash curler beforehand.
- We then made a custom lip color for Hana's lips using Etude House Play 101 Pencils (told ya they were versatile). We started off by filling her entire lips with shade #22, and then went over it with the dark brown shade #50.

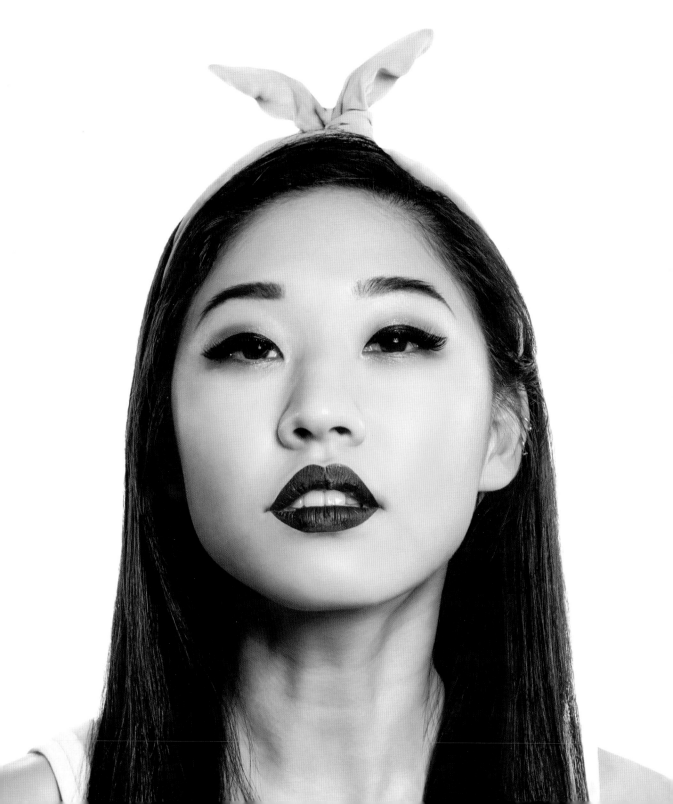

We loved this look so much we wanted to show it on a variety of women. Here we have the beautiful Lanny, Kelly, and Amelia all rockin' the Bad Girl look, joined by their bad boy Rich.

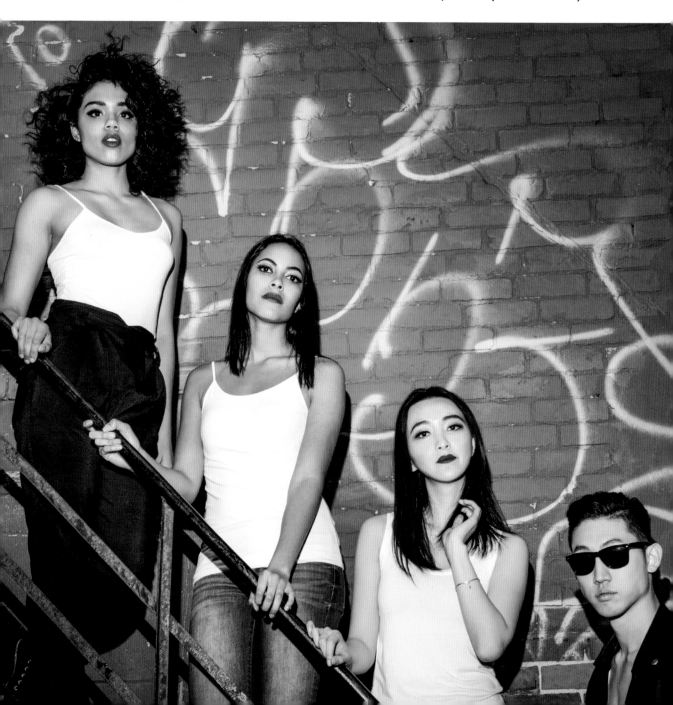

PUPPY EYE VS. CAT EYE

The cat eye has reigned supreme since the days of the pharaohs, and it's a cute look—it's stuck around for a reason. But sometimes your eye shape just won't allow for a good cat eye, or maybe you'd just like to branch out and try something a little different. If either of those is the case, why not give the puppy eye a try? The only difference between the two is the puppy eye has a slight downtick whereas the cat eye has a slight uptick. You may think that by sloping your eyeliner down it's going to make for a drowsy look, but just the opposite is true. The puppy eye elongates and widens the eyes, giving them a rounder, more alert look.

- To get this look, line your upper lid as normal. Then go back in and start at the middle of your eye and work your way out, following the downward curve of your eye and extending a bit beyond it.
- Then bring your liner down to your lower lashes, creating a triangle shape. Fill in the triangle and there you have it, a puppy eye!

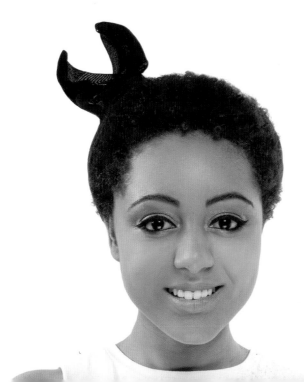

SWEET RED BEAN

My makeup is often inspired by things around me, and apparently I'm surrounded by a lot of snacks. Here we have another look inspired by an old-fashioned Korean treat. When I first opened the eyeliner that was the basis of this look, it immediately made me think of the deep red color you see when you bite into *gyeongju* bread. *Gyeongju* bread is a cute little pastry cake filled with a sweet red bean paste. Here Lanny is serving you some serious red bean smolder.

- We started off by prepping her skin with a mist of Whamisa Organic Flowers Damask Rose Petal Mist, a hydrating mist with ingredients better than most toners.
- We then applied a 3:1 mixture of VDL Lumilayer Primer with Dr. Jart+ Premium Beauty Balm SPF 45 in Light to Medium all over her face.
- Her eyebrows were filled into a straight shape with The Face Shop Brow Master Eyebrow Kit in 02 Grey Brown.
- I patted on Etude House Proof 10 Primer on her lids and then our makeup artist Chloe brushed 3 Concept Eyes Gel Eye Liner in the shade Love all over Lanny's lids. She then smudged it out with her fingers and patted on Etude House Look At My Eyes Cafe eyeshadow PK004 Deep Berry Soda to really enhance the deep red-bean color.
- Next, she tightlined the upper and lower eyelids with TonyMoly Backstage Gel Eyeliner in Black. She then used the same liner to draw a thick line on the upper lid, winging it out into a soft puppy eye. She then quickly blended the thick line on the lids before it set so that it softly faded into the eyeshadow.
- For extra oomph we topped her TonyMoly Delight Circle Lens Mascara No.1 Volume Circle coated lashes with a pair of false eyelashes. We didn't want to take the focus away from the eyes so we kept blush and lipstick to a nude minimum, sweeping Innisfree Mineral Shading #7 Sweet Vanilla on the cheeks, topping it with Innisfree Mineral Glow Stick Highlighter around the C-zones, and finishing the whole thing off with TonyMoly Kiss Lover Style Lip Stick #BE03 Coco Beige (sidenote: I would be lying if I said I didn't initially buy this lipstick because it has my name on it, haaa).

All together this made for one incredibly delicious look.

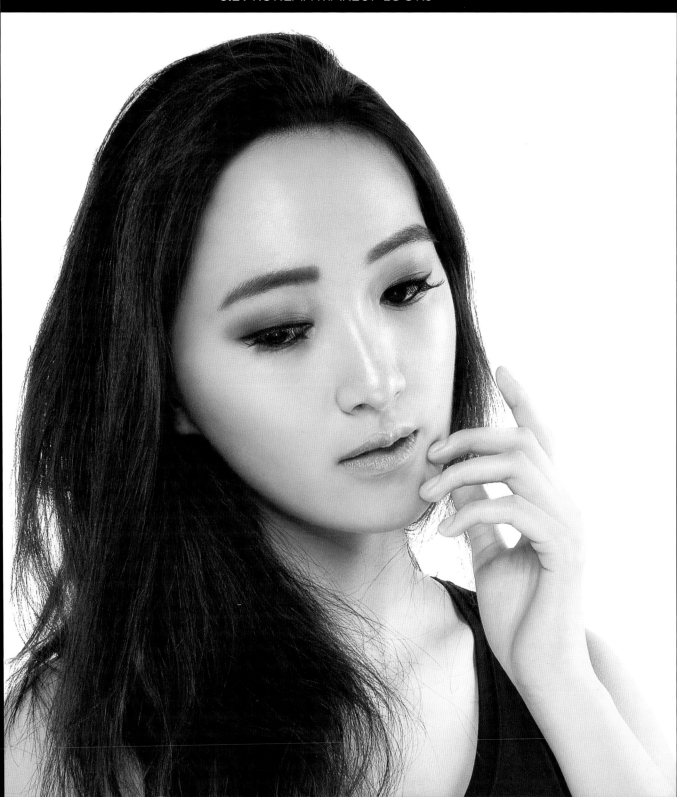

BAE BAE

There is a K-pop video that my daughter has become obsessed with, it's filled with lots of gorgeous purples, bronzes, and pink colors throughout. After being made to watch it for about the fiftieth time, I finally gave in to its charms. From there, the video's color palette stuck with me when it came time to go to the studio and shoot the looks for this book. Lea, our hazel-eyed beauty, was who I thought of immediately for this look.

- Lea's skin was prepped with spritzes of Whamisa Organic Flowers Olive Leaf Mist and Innisfree Mineral Moisture Fitting Base.
- I then applied Innisfree Eco Natural Green Tea BB Cream in shade 01.
- Her brows were filled with The Face Shop Brow Master Eyebrow Kit in 01 Beige Brown.
- I gave our makeup artist Chloe the Pony x Memebox Shine Easy Glam Eyeshadow Palette #1 and asked her to give Lea a smoky eye using the sparkling shades in the right side of the palette (the shadows on the left side has matte finishes). She used the colors Shine Gold and Glam Cocoa to give her a bronzy, shimmering look. Shine Gold was used all over the eye top and bottom and Glam Cocoa was used around the outer corners of the lower lids and softly blended into the crease. Shine Rosegold was used in the teardrop highlight.
- Her lash line was tightlined and her waterline was filled in with Etude House Play 101 Pencil in shade #50.
- TonyMoly Backstage Gel Eyeliner in Black was used to line the lids and a pair of false eyelashes were attached.
- Highlighter was applied with Innisfree Mineral Glow Stick on the C-zone, forehead, and cupid's bow.
- We gave her a sweet pink flush with The Face Shop Soft Cream Blusher in 01 Pink.
- What really makes this look exquisite is the blazing orchid shade on her lips, which was provided with my favorite lipstick in one of my favorite shades, VDL Expert Color Lip Cube in #301 Night Orchid.

When this gorgeous purple is paired with the shimmering bronze eye, it's enough to make you pass every reflective surface you can find so that you might admire how stunning you look.

Hey, bae bae! Would you like a little sweet red bean?

BLUSHING EYES

Much like George Costanza leaving the room on a high note, I'd like to leave you on this daring note. This look takes a fair amount of courage to pull-off, but once you try it, I promise you'll like it. Even our model Hue-Linh gave me a look when I told her what we were about to do to her face, but her smile once we showed her our handiwork said it all. This look is called Blushing Eyes because we completely forgo cheek blush and leave it to the eyes to carry this look with a soft, unexpected, daring flush.

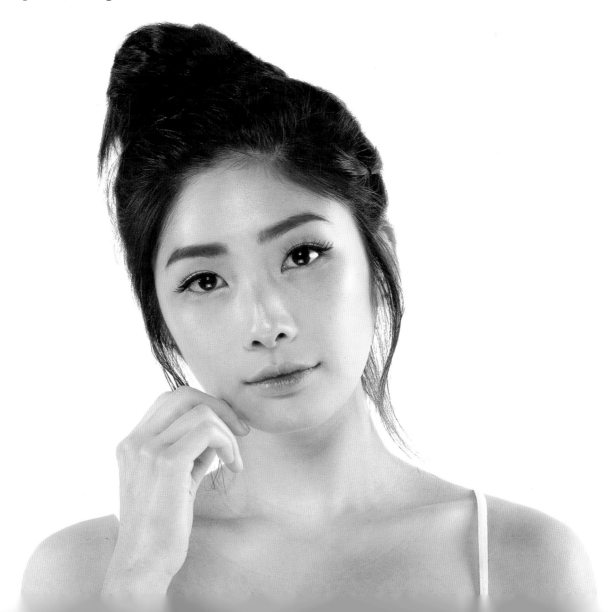

- First we prepped the skin with Nature Republic Bee Venom Mist Essence.
- We then applied VDL Lumilayer Primer all over her face followed by the Innisfree Water Glow Cushion in #23.
- Her eyebrows were filled with The Face Shop Brow Master Eyebrow Kit in 01 Beige Brown and then topped with Holika Holika Wonder Drawing 1 Sec. Finish Browcara in #4 Dark Brown.
- The eyes of this look are similar to what she wore for the soft gradient look, however this time we used VDL Expert Color Eye Book 6.4. #01. Shade Pantone 7515 Caramelize was patted all over the the lid and crease.
- A soft cat eye was applied with Clio Waterproof Pen Liner Kill Black, followed up with a coating of It's Skin Babyface Mascara 02 Volume Setting Black.
- We then added some glamour by applying a pair of false demi eyelashes to the outer corners of her lids.
- Her lower lids are kept soft, we skipped lower lash mascara and Clio Gelpresso Waterproof Pencil Shadow in #1 Make Me Up as a highlight was used in place of bottom eyeliner.
- Our makeup artist, Chloe, then used a very light, delicate hand to brush on the shade Pantone 18-1438 Marsala under the eyes, extending ever so slightly out beyond the orbital bone. The VLD + Pantone Expert Color Eye Book 6.4 is a limited edition product, but there are similar shades to be found in the TonyMoly Eyetone eyeshadow line if you can't get your hands on one.
- We wanted the lips to echo the eyes, so we did a delicate gradient lip. To keep the softness going, we started with a generous coat of Whamisa Organic Flowers Lip Moisture and topped that with Clio Tension Lip in shade 09 Pinkvely.

The soft luminous skin, unexpected uses of classic products, and innovative formulations really brings together everything I love about K-beauty. This look both symbolizes and sums up the source of my enthusiasm, and why I think K-beauty is so incredible. Korean beauty is truly extraordinary and we invite you to get on board with us and join our never-ending adventure through this thrilling industry. We thank you so much for coming with us on this journey!

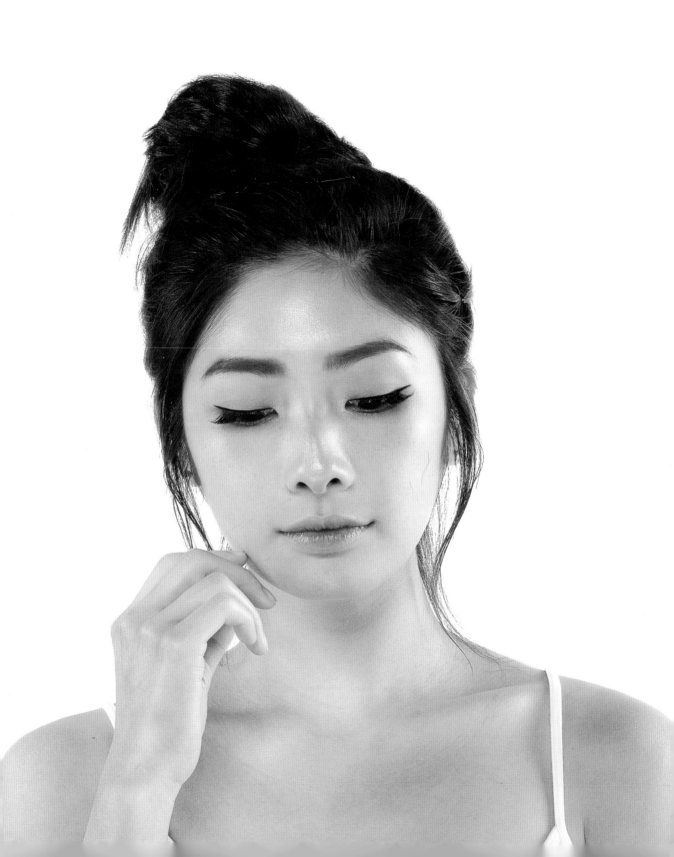

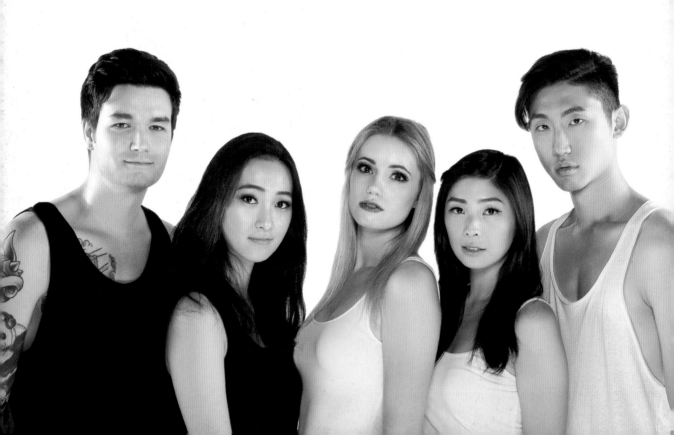

PART 4
ADDITIONAL RESOURCES

Okay, now for the best part: shopping! It's time to get out there and start searching for your new favorite Korean beauty products. There are a *huge* number of K-beauty shopping options out there, so we've assembled this guide as a starting point for your retail adventures.

We've also made the assumption that you love a good deal just as much as we do, so we've set up a website at kerryandcoco.com, where you can find a frequently updated list of exclusive coupons and discount referral codes for a growing list of Korean cosmetics sellers, including Glow Recipe, Wishtrend, W2Beauty, and more.

U.S. BASED ONLINE BOUTIQUES

These boutiques are all U.S. based, and most of them ship to Canada, United Kingdom, and Australia, as well. They each offer their own selection of Korean brands and products, which are chosen based on the retailer's individual philosophy and approach to beauty and skincare.

Glow Recipe	glowrecipe.com
Insider Beauty	insiderbeauty.com
Peach & Lily	peachandlily.com
Pretty & Cute	prettyandcute.com
Soko Glam	sokoglam.com

MAINSTREAM U.S. STORES

These are major retailers with a large presence in the United States, and in some cases, worldwide. These stores carry at least one Korean line of products, and in many cases, more. Visit kerryandcoco.com to see a current list of Korean brands available though each of these retailers.

Bloomingdales	bloomingdales.com
Forever21	forever21.com
Neiman Marcus	neimanmarcus.com
Nordstrom	nordstrom.com
Sephora	sephora.com
Target	target.com
Urban Outfitters	urbanoutfitters.com

KOREAN BRANDS WITH INTERNATIONAL WEBSITES

Many Korean brands have an online presence that caters to international customers. These brand websites are tailored toward the United States, and many also ship to Canada, United Kingdom., and Australia.

3 Concept Eyes	en.stylenanda.com
Amorepacific	us.amorepacific.com
Chosunguh	en.chosungah22.com
Club Clio USA	clubcliousa.com

Etude House	etudehouse.com
Innisfree	innisfreeworld.com
Missha	misshaus.com
	missha.com.au
	missha.co.nz
Moonshot	en.moonshot-cosmetics.com
Sulwhasoo	us.sulwhasoo.com
The Face Shop	thefaceshop-america.com
	thefaceshopwa.com.au
	thefaceshop.co.nz
TonyMoly	TonyMolyus.com

KOREAN SHOPS WITH INTERNATIONAL SHIPPING

These online retailers are based out of South Korea. They offer the widest variety of product selection and international shipping choices. Most of these shops will ship to nearly anywhere in the world, and for many locations, there are expedited shipping options available that can get your purchases from Seoul to your front door in less than a week!

Korea Depart	en.koreadepart.com
RoseRoseShop	roseroseshop.com

Jolse	jolse.com
W2Beauty	w2beauty.com
Wishtrend	wishtrend.com

KOREAN MARKETPLACES & SHOPPING SERVICES

These shopping options are for the advanced K-beauty explorers. 11st & Gmarket are huge online market places with hundreds of sellers, and offer brands that may be difficult to find anywhere else at prices as low as (or close to) what you'd pay for them in South Korea. Avecko is a shopping service that will procure goods from any Korean shopping site and ship them to you. All of these options have a variety of international shipping options. They're a great way to score some great deals on Korean brands you already love, or find some new, under-the-radar K-beauty treasures!

11st	english.11st.co.kr
Avecko	avecko.com
Gmarket	global.gmarket.co.kr

EBAY & AMAZON

There are many Korean cosmetics sellers on eBay and on Amazon. In fact, Amazon even has an entire storefront dedicated to Korean beauty products! Both of these marketplaces are worth exploring, but be vigilant—there is also a large number of sellers that are stocking and selling counterfeit and expired products, sometimes even without the seller's knowledge. It's important to look for sellers that have a lot of feedback, and who also have an average positive feedback score of 97% or higher. You can also visit kerryandcoco.com for an extensive list of reliable eBay and Amazon sellers.

COMMON INGREDIENT COMPONENTS

English	Korean
Acid	애씨드
Alcohol	알코올
Extract	추출물
Ferment	발효
Leaf	잎
Oil	오일
Root	뿌리
Seed	씨앗

Some Korean products include product ingredient information in English, but many do not. If you have specific ingredient sensitivities or preferences, it can be helpful to know what the Korean translation is. In this ingredient glossary, you'll find English-Korean translations for nearly 250 cosmetic ingredients.

2-ethylhexyl p-methoxycinnamate	2- 에칠헥실 p-메톡시신나메이트
3-(4-Methyl benzylidene) camphor	3-(4-메틸 벤질리덴) 캠퍼
Alcohol	알코올
Allantoin	알란토인
Allium Sativum (Garlic) Bulb Extract	마늘추출물
Almond Oil	아몬드 오일
Aloe Vera	알로에 베라
Amino Acids / Peptides	아미노산 / 펩타이드
Ammonium Lauryl Sulfate	암모늄라우릴설페이트
Anise Oil	아니스 오일
Apricot Oil	살구씨 오일
Arbutin	알부틴
Argan Oil	아르간 오일
Arginine	알지닌
Ascorbyl Tetraisopalmitate	아스코빌 테트라이소팔미테이트
Asparagus Cochinchinensis Root Extract	천문동추출물
Astragalus Membranaceus Root Extract	황기추출물
Atractyloides Japonica Root Oil	백출 오일
Avobenzone	아보벤존
Azealic Acid	아젤라익애씨드
Bee Venom	벌독
Beeswax	비즈왁스

Bemotrizinol	베모트리지놀
Benzophenone-3	벤조페논-3
Beta-Glucan	베타-글루칸
Betaine	베타인
Betaine Salicylate	베타인 살리실레이트
Bifida Ferment Lysate	비피다 발효 용해물
Birch oil extract	자작나무 오일 추출물
Bird's Nest	제비집
Bis-Ethylhexyloxyphenol Methoxyphenyl Triazine	비스-에칠헥실옥시페놀메톡시페닐트리아진
Black Sugar	흑설탕
Butyl-methoxydibenzoilmethane	부틸-메톡시디벤조일메탄
Butylene Glycol	부틸렌글라이콜
Butylparaben	부틸파라벤
Caffeine	카페인
Camellia Oil	동백 오일
Camellia Sinensis	녹차
Caprylyl/Capryl Glucoside	카프릴릴/카프릴글루코사이드
Carbolic Acid	페놀(석탄산)
Carbomer	카보머
Caviar / Salmon Egg	캐비어 / 연어알
Centella Asiatica (Gotu Kola)	병풀 (고투 콜라)

Ceramides	세라마이드
Cetearyl Alcohol	세테아릴알코올
Cetyl Alcohol	세틸 알코올
Charcoal	숯
Cheese	치즈
Chestnut Oil	밤 오일
Chrysanthellum Indicum Extract	감국추출물
Citric Acid	시트릭애씨드
Citrus Unshiu Peel Extract	귤껍질추출물
Clay	클레이
Cnidium Officinale Root Extract	천궁추출물
Cocamidopropyl Betaine	코카미도프로필베타인
Coco-Glucoside	코코-글루코사이드
Cocoa Butter	코코아 버터
Coconut Oil	코코넛 오일
Collagen	콜라겐
Coptis Chinensis Root Extract	황련추출물
Cordyceps Militaris Extract	밀리타리스동충하초추출물
Cordyceps Sinensis Extract	동충하초 추출물
Cucumber Extract	오이 추출물
Cyclohexasiloxane	사이클로헥사실록산

Cyclomethicone	사이클로메치콘
Decyl Glucoside	데실글루코사이드
Deer Antler Extract	녹용 추출물
Denatured Alcohol	변성알코올
Diethylamino hydroxybenzoyl hexyl benzoate	디에칠아미노 하이드록시벤조일 헥실 벤조에이트
Dimethicone	디메치콘
Dioscorea Villosa (Wild Yam) Root Extract	야생얌뿌리추출물
Disodium Cocoamphodiacetate	디소듐코코암포디아세테이트
Disodium EDTA	디소듐이디티에이
Disodium Lauryl Sulfosuccinate	디소듐라우릴설포석시네이트
Donkey Milk	당나귀유
Egg Yolk	난황
Emu Oil	에뮤 오일
Ethanol	에탄올
Ethyl Alcohol	에틸알코올
Ethylhexyl Methoxycinnamate	에칠헥실메톡시신나메이트
Ethylhexyl Salicate	에틸헥실살리실레이트
Ethylhexyl Triazone	에틸헥실트리아존
Ethylhexyldimethyl-p-Aminobenzoate	에틸헥실디메틸-P-아미노벤조에이트
Evening Primrose Oil	달맞이꽃 오일
Ferulic Acid	페룰릭애씨드

Fragrance	향료
Ghassoul Clay	가슬 클레이
Ginkgo Biloba Leaf Extract	은행잎추출물
Ginkgo Biloba Nut Extract	은행추출물
Glycerides	글리세라이드
Glycerin	글리세린
Glycerol	글리세롤
Glycine Soja (Soybean) Oil	콩 오일(콩기름)
Glycol Stearate	글라이콜스테아레이트
Glycolic Acid	글라이콜릭애씨드
Glycyrrhiza Glabra (Licorice) Root	감초
Goat Milk	산양유
Grapefruit Extract	자몽 추출물
Grapeseed Oil	포도씨 오일
Green Clay	그린 클레이
Green Tea	녹차
Helianthus Annuus (Sunflower) Seed Oil	해바라기씨오일
Hexylene Glycol	헥실렌글라이콜
Honey	꿀
Honeysuckle Extract	인동덩굴추출물
Horse Oil	마유

Hyaluronic Acid	히알루로닉애씨드
Hydrogenated Vegetable Oil	하이드로제네이티드식물성오일
Isoamyl p-Methoxycinnamate	이소아밀 p-메톡시신나메이트
Isopropyl Alcohol	이소프로필알코올
Jojoba Oil	호호바 오일
L Ascorbic Acid	아스코빅애씨드
Lactic Acid	락틱애씨드
Lactobacillus Ferment	락토바실러스발효물
Lanolin	라놀린
Lauryl Glucoside	라우릴글루코사이드
Lauryl Phosphate	라우릴포스페이트
Lecithin	레시틴
Lemon Extract	레몬추출물
Licorice Root	감초 뿌리
Limnanthes Alba Seed Oil	메도우폼씨오일
Linoleic Acid	리놀레익애씨드
Lycium Chinense Extract	구기자나무추출물
Macadamia Oil	마카다미아 오일
Macadamia Seed Oil	마카다미아씨오일
Malic Acid	말릭애씨드
Mango Seed Butter	망고씨 버터

Meadowfoam Seed Oil	메도우폼씨 오일
Methanol	메탄올
Methyl Methacrylate Crosspolymer	메칠메타크릴레이트크로스폴리머
Methylparaben	메칠파라벤
Mica	마이카
Mineral Oil	미네랄 오일
Mink Oil	밍크 오일
Momordica Charantia Fruit Extract	여주열매추출물
Morus Alba Extract	뽕나무추출물
Mugwort Extract	쑥추출물
Mulberry Extract	오디 추출물
Myristyl Myristate	미리스틸 미리스테이트
Natto Gum	낫토검
Nelumbo Nucifera Leaf (Lotus) Extract	연꽃잎추출물
Niacinamide	니코틴산아미드
Octocrylene	옥토크릴린
Oleic Acid	올레익애씨드
Oligopeptide	올리고펩타이드
Olive Oil	올리브 오일
Ophiopogon Japonicus Root Extract	맥문동 추출물
Orchid Extract	난추출물

Oryza Sativa Extract	쌀 추출물
Paeonia Lactiflora Root Extract	작약 추출물
Panax Ginseng	인삼
Panax Ginseng Root Extract	인삼추출물
Panthenol	판테놀
Paraben	파라벤
Paraffin	파라핀
Passionfruit Oil	패션후르츠 오일
Pearl Extract	진주추출물
PEG-100 Stearate	PEG-100 스테아레이트
Pentylene Glycol	펜틸렌글라이콜
Petroleum	페트롤리움
Phenol	페놀
Phenoxyethanol	페녹시에탄올
Phenyl Trimethicone	페닐 트리메치콘
Pig Collagen	돼지 콜라겐
Placenta	태반
Polydextrose	폴리덱스트로오스
Polygonum Multiflorum Root Extract	하수오 추출물
Polyisobutane	폴리이소부텐
Polypeptide	폴리펩타이드

Polysorbate 20	폴리소르베이트 20
Polysorbate 80	폴리소르베이트 80
Pomegranate Oil	석류 오일
Potassium Hydroxide	포타슘하이드록사이드
Potassium Lauryl Sulfate	포타슘라우릴설페이트
Potassium Sorbate	포타슘소르베이트
Propanediol	프로판디올
Propolis	프로폴리스
Propylene Glycol	프로필렌글라이콜
Pure Gold	순금
Raspberry Extract	라즈베리 추출물
Red Ginseng	홍삼
Retinal	레티날
Retinaldehyde	레틴알데하이드
Retinoid	레티노이드
Retinol	레티놀
Retinyl Palmitate	레티닐 팔미테이트
Rice Bran Extract	쌀겨 추출물
Rose Oil	장미 오일
Rosehip Oil	로즈힙 오일
Rosemary Extract	로즈마리 추출물

Royal Jelly	로얄젤리
Saccharomyces Ferment	효모 발효물
Safflower Seed Oil	홍화씨 오일
Salicylic Acid	살리실릭애씨드
Salvia Hispanica Seed Extract	치아씨 추출물
Saponins	사포닌
Schizandra Chinensis Fruit Extract	오미자 추출물
SD Alcohol	SD 알코올
Sesame Oil	참깨오일
Shea Butter	시어 버터
Silica	실리카
Silicone	실리콘
Snail Ferment Filtrate	달팽이 발효 여과물
Snail Mucin	달팽이 점액
Snail Secretion Filtrate	달팽이점액여과물
Sodium Benzoate	소듐벤조에이트
Sodium Cocoyl Isethionate	소듐코코일이세치오네이트
Sodium Dodecyl Sulfate	소듐도데실설페이트
Sodium Hyaluronate	소듐하이알루로네이트
Sodium Hydroxide	소듐하이드록사이드
Sodium Laureth Sulfate	소듐라우레스설페이트

Sodium Lauroyl Isethionate	소듐 라우로일 이세치오네이트
Sodium Lauryl Sulfate	소듐 라우릴 설페이트
Sodium Myreth Sulfate	소듐미레스설페이트
Sodium Polyacrylate	소듐폴리아크릴레이트
Sorbitol	소르비톨
Soybean Extract	대두 추출물
Soybean Ferment Extract	대두 발효 추출물
Soybean Sprout Extract	콩나물 추출물
Squalane	스쿠알란
Squalene	스쿠알렌
Starfish Extract	불가사리 추출물
Stearic Acid	스테아릭애씨드
Sugar	설탕
Syn-ake	씨네이크
Tea Tree Oil	티트리 오일
Terminalia Chebula Root Extract	가자나무추출물
Theobroma Cacao (Cocoa)	카카오
Titanium Dioxide	티타늄디옥사이드
Tocopheryl	토코페릴
Tocopheryl Acetate	토코페릴 아세테이트
Trehalose	트레할로스

Triclosan	트리클로산
Triethyoxycaprylylsilane	트리에톡시카프릴릴실란
Triglycerides	트리글리세라이드
Trimethylsiloxysilicate	트리메칠실록시실리케이트
Tris-Biphenyl Triazine	트리스-비페닐 트라이진
Urea	우레아
Volcanic Ash	화산재
Water	물
Wild Ginseng Extract	산삼 추출물
Willow Bark	버드나무 껍질
Willow Bark Extract	버드나무 추출물
Xylitol	자일리톨
Yeast Ferment	효모발효
Yeast Ferment Extract	효모발효추출물
Yogurt	요구르트
Zinc Oxide	징크옥사이드

ACKNOWLEDGMENTS

Many people helped make this book possible, but we would like to specially thank:

Chloe Kaypee, for her hard work and amazing makeup skills. We were so lucky to find you, and we can't wait to work with you again in the future.

Rebeca Alfonzo, for being our last-minute photography savior, and for all of her photo correcting wizardry.

Pedram Navid, for trekking out to Montreal and shooting an amazing book cover.

Amélie Mcgarrell, Sarah Vega, Marlond Samedy, Laureen Pressoir, Kelly Hennegen, Lea Roth, Lanny Lou, Huh-Linh Tran, Richard Park, and Hana Park for being such amazing, hard-working, beautiful, and patient models.

Cat, Tracy, Elisa, Sheryll, Jude, Ryan, and Rebecca for contributing such incredible, detailed skincare routines.

Alice and Eddie, for all of their input on Korean brands and beauty trends.

Celeste JO, for her expertise in assisting with the ingredient translations.

CREDITS

PHOTOGRAPHY
Rebeca Alfonzo and Pedram Navid

MAKEUP
Coco Park and Chloe Kaypee

PHOTOGRAPHIC ART DIRECTION
Coco Park

COVER DESIGN
Kerry Thompson and Coco Park

BOOK LAYOUT & DESIGN
Kerry Thompson

PHOTO CREDITS

REBECA ALFONZO

Back cover, pages 4, 12, 18, 195, 196, 200, 202, 203, 204, 205, 207, 209, 211, 212, 213, 215, 217, 219, 221, 222, 223, 225, 226

PEDRAM NAVID

Front cover, pages 199, 215, 216

BLOGGER PHOTO CREDITS

MODELS

KELLY HENNEGEN
Page 216

LANNY LOU
Front cover, pages 199, 219,
222, 226

AMÉLIE MCGARRELL
Front cover, pages 197, 199, 216

HANA PARK
Page 215

RICHARD PARK
Pages 4, 158, 196, 212, 216, 226

LAUREEN PRESSOIR
Pages 197, 217

LEA ROTH
Back cover, pages 200, 212,
221, 222, 226

MARLOND SAMEDY
Pages 4, 18

CHASE STRAIGHT
Page 226

HUH-LINH TRAN
Back cover, pages 12, 202,
203, 204, 205, 207, 211,
223, 225, 226

SARAH VEGA
Back cover, pages 195, 196,
209, 212, 213